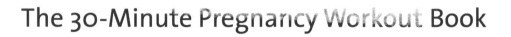

The 30-Minute Pregnancy Workout Book

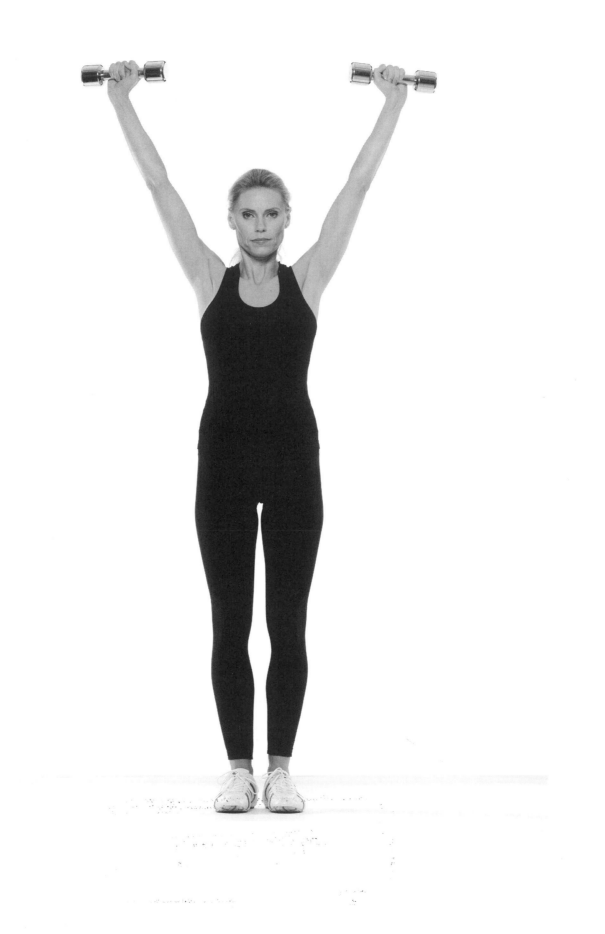

The 30-Minute Pregnancy Workout Book

The Complete Light Weight Program for Fitness

Anna Aberg

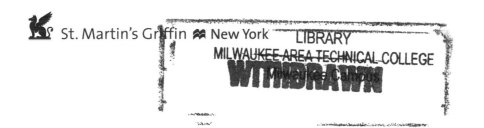

St. Martin's Griffin ❧ New York

THE 30-MINUTE PREGNANCY WORKOUT BOOK. Copyright © 2008 by Anna Aberg. All rights reserved. Printed in the United States of America. For information, address St. Martin's Press, 175 Fifth Avenue, New York, N.Y. 10010.

www.stmartins.com

Photographs copyright © 2008 by Ralf Ekvall

Book design and composition by Gretchen Achilles

Library of Congress Cataloging-in-Publication Data
Aberg, Anna.
    The 30-minute pregnancy workout book : the complete light weight program for fitness /
Anna Aberg.—1st ed.
        p. cm.
    ISBN-13: 978-0-312-37282-8
    ISBN-10: 0-312-37282-5
  1. Physical fitness for pregnant women. 2. Exercise for pregnant women. I. Title.
    RG558.7.A24 2008
    618.2'44—dc22   2008012432

First Edition: July 2008

10 9 8 7 6 5 4 3 2 1

Thank you all for being part of the creations of my life,

but I don't owe anybody my spirit.

I have the right to care for myself and my loved ones.

I cherish your unconditional respect and affection.

I have chosen not to live my life to prove myself as I realize that life is never

perfect, and despite life's limitations, I am nourished by everyone's love,

and for that I am truly grateful.

Contents

Acknowledgments

I feel so fortunate to be able to share the following experiences. They could not have come about without the help and support of some special people in my life.

Thank you:

To my editor, Elizabeth Beier, whose enormous guidance and input I could not have done without. My gratitude to you, Elizabeth.

To Michelle Richter, thank you for your patience and help as another important team member. And, of course, to all those at St. Martin's Press.

To the man in my life, my soul mate, my life partner, Paul Anka, who is always there and gives me wings to fly. Thank you. I am so lucky to have you and our son, Ethan, and my daughter, Elli, in my life.

To Ethan and Elli—for the love, joy, and pleasure that you bring into my life: I could not ask for more.

To Steven Cohen, for your support and belief.

To my attorney, Stuart Silfen, for making this possible, and to Jill Erickson, whose professionalism and caring I so admire.

Special thanks to Tony Lofaro for being there.

To my mentors, Jerzy and Angela Gregorek and Johnny G. Thank you for opening my eyes to the world of Olympic Training. And, Johnny, thank you for teaching me the connection between the mind and the body.

I want to thank Dr. Katz for delivering two healthy and beautiful babies, and for his ongoing support for the contents of this book. His generous and compassionate words, "I have never seen a fitter mom than you, Anna," are ones that I cherish.

To Ralf Ekvall, the greatest photographer I ever worked with. Thank you for the contribution.

Last, to Julie Zhu, Bessy Wong, Jackie Cruz, Madeleine Larsson, Suss Erlandsson, Cecilia Palmqvist, Jessica Malmlof, Lotta Lilja, for your understanding and for always being there.

About Anna Aberg

Anna Aberg grew up in a small farming town in southern Sweden, far from the bright lights of Los Angeles, where she has made her mark in the fitness industry as an athlete, personal trainer, fitness model, and now author of the new exercise book for pregnant women, *The 30-Minute Pregnancy Workout Book.*

Sweden prides itself on its very fit citizens; however, physical fitness was not always of interest to Aberg. The avid horseback rider and basketball player dreamed of becoming a scientist, even while her parents steered her to get an economics degree instead. Aberg was nevertheless determined to follow her own path to success. At fifteen, she moved to Helsingborg, Sweden's fourth-largest city, to study at a university. She also got a part-time job as a UPS driver, quickly proving she could be as tough as male drivers when she began to strap two-pound weights to her legs during her delivery rounds.

A chance stop on her delivery route at the Nautilus Company led her to meet owner Mats Thulin, who was impressed by Aberg's growing enthusiasm for exercise equipment and physical fitness. She completed Thulin's training program and became one of his company's instructors, teaching people how to properly use the exercise machines. A modeling career followed when Aberg was eighteen, and her sleek physique was soon appearing on billboards, advertisements, and commercials.

In 1994, Aberg was named Miss Sweden, Miss Hawaiian Tropic, and later Miss Fitness of Scandinavia, a contest sponsored by Nautilus. Those titles gave her an opportunity to visit the United States for the first time in 1995 to compete in Miss Hawaiian Tropic International, where she placed among the top ten. That experience led her to her calling as a personal trainer and fitness guru.

Aberg moved to Los Angeles and met Johnny G, a trainer and endurance athlete who developed the Spinning stationary bike program. She became an instructor and a spokeswoman for his fitness business. Aberg earned her certificate as a fitness trainer, taught Spinning classes to Sharon Stone, and worked at Crunch, one of Los Angeles's most popular gyms. She also trained Paul Marciano of Guess, Inc.; Tracee Ross, daughter of Diana Ross; and investment banker Brad Freeman.

Aberg's growing reputation in the fitness industry launched her work with some of the big names in the business, including Olympic weight lifter Jerzy Gregorek and Greg Isaacs, author of *The Ultimate Lean Routine*. She also had film and television roles in *The Specialist* with Sylvester Stallone, *Drop Zone* with Wesley Snipes, *Bio-Dome, Dumb & Dumber,* and *Baywatch*. As a personal trainer, she was also a featured fitness model in *Fitness* magazine, *Shape, Health & Fitness, Natural Health, Sports Fitness,* as well as *Elle, Mode,* and *Harper's Bazaar*.

Her knowledge, experience, and extensive training prepared her to write about the techniques she learned in the fitness industry. *The 30-Minute Pregnancy Workout Book* is a simple-to-follow guide for women who are eager to understand the body changes that occur during pregnancy. The book will teach women how to stay fit and healthy during this exciting yet challenging period of their adult lives.

When Aberg learned she was going to have a baby, she became concerned about how best to stay fit during the nine months of pregnancy. Aberg—who is now mother to Elli, five, and Ethan, two and a half—had only 11 percent body fat when she was pregnant, and that rose to 15 percent when she gave birth. Her weight gain during her pregnancy was only sixteen pounds, and seven of those pounds were from the baby.

The workout book will show pregnant women how to train properly, without necessarily visiting a gym to perform the exercises shown. It is a full-body training program using weights to give women a good cardio workout. The exercises focus on flexibility, speed, and power, and on the little ligaments and small muscles in the body. It can be done in thirty minutes.

Aberg, who is five feet eight inches and 120 pounds, has trained vigorously for twenty years. She is determined, enjoys challenges, and wants to show women that keeping up with their fitness during pregnancy is nothing to be scared about. It can be done safely, with the right exercises and in consultation with a doctor.

"I've come to realize when you work out, you want to maintain the youthfulness of your body. It's what we're all looking for," says Aberg.

Foreword

When Anna Aberg was pregnant with her first child, everyone told her she would lose her slim figure and gain extra weight no matter what she did. Aberg, a fitness guru ever since moving to the United States from her native Sweden in the mid-nineties, was determined to prove them wrong.

The result is *The 30-Minute Pregnancy Workout Book*, a fascinating book designed exclusively for women, particularly expectant mothers. In its easy-to-follow and straightforward format, it will help you achieve ultimate fitness during pregnancy by combining a simple program that uses free weights and regular exercises to gain flexibility and strength in your body. It will help many women achieve their ultimate goal: being lean and strong. The beauty of Aberg's program is that the exercises described take a mere thirty minutes. Anybody can spare half an hour a day to look and feel wonderful.

Make this routine a gift to yourself, your partner—and your future child. Aberg knows what she's talking about. She comes from Sweden, a Scandinavian country that prides itself on having a population of healthy citizens. She's been in the fitness industry for twenty years as a personal trainer in Los Angeles, where she worked with endurance-athlete trainers and Olympic weight lifters, taught Spinning classes, and even trained Hollywood celebrities such as Sharon Stone.

While pregnant with her two children, Elli and Ethan, Aberg practiced the exercises she created for the book and got amazing results. Remarkably, she was able to go through a strong, healthy pregnancy with only a 4-percent increase in body fat.

"The whole purpose of this book is to show women how to train, and that you don't have to go to the gym; everything can be done in your home. The program only takes thirty minutes a day, five times a week," says Aberg, who has modeled as well as appeared in movies and commercials since she moved to the United States.

There are all kinds of fitness books on the market, but nothing matches Aberg's unique take on how to work your body. This specially crafted exercise program combines strength and flexibility to work the entire body and doesn't just focus on individual muscle groups. Aberg's program uses exercises that will give you a complete functional workout without relying on single repetitions that can often strain joints and ligaments. Her program is special and delivers an overall-conditioning knockout punch.

Aberg feels strongly that expectant mothers should take proper care of their bodies. She says it's important that a pregnant woman eat nutritious foods and exercise on a regular basis in order to establish a good pattern for her unborn baby.

The fitness and diet business is a multi-billion-dollar industry in the United States, largely supported by big marketing campaigns that strive to convince people that they will feel good about themselves if they use their products. "Fitness should help people; it shouldn't just be used to make money," says Aberg, who has a passion for people taking responsibility for their health and well-being.

It's all about personal choice, says Aberg. "Nobody is forcing you to eat fast food or watch TV five hours a night instead of exercising." Perfect for women of all ages and body types, *The 30-Minute Pregnancy Workout Book* can be the first step toward achieving a truly healthy lifestyle.

Try it: Your body will thank you!

—TONY LOFARO, April 2008
Tony Lofaro is a reporter with the *Ottawa Citizen*,
a daily newspaper in Ottawa, Canada.

A Note to Readers

Pregnant women should always check with their doctor before attempting any kind of exercise program. Some types of exercises and their frequency could be too strenuous for some pregnant women. If a woman is fit and healthy before becoming pregnant, exercise is less likely to be risky. The risks are greater for women who have had a previous injury or who have a preexisting condition. When performing an exercise, if you become nauseated or unsteady on your feet, you should stop. If you experience any kind of uneasiness, exercise should be discontinued at once.

The 30-Minute Pregnancy Workout Book

Introduction

Congratulations! You're pregnant. (Even if you're not, you can keep reading.)

How many pregnancy books have you looked at so far? Ten? Twenty? Can you even remember at this point? You might just be glancing at this one in a bookstore. Perhaps it's one of those really nice stores where they have armchairs arranged for you to sit awhile and read. There are a lot of books in this store, but the one you're holding is a little different. I looked at dozens of books when I was pregnant, too. Maybe even hundreds. Books, magazines, Web pages, newspaper articles—I read anything I could find. I'd never had a baby before, and it seemed like there was so much to learn. There were so many changes going on in my body, and in the little body growing inside me, and I was determined to find information on those changes, and what they meant for me.

I encountered hundreds of books designed to educate, support, and comfort women during pregnancy; a few yoga books; some Pilates workbooks; and one or two huge volumes that read like technical manuals. I was disappointed to find that nobody had written a book about having a *healthy pregnancy,* a guide that could answer simple questions about the exercises I was already doing. Like, is it important to exercise during pregnancy? Should I still do abdominal exercises? Did I need to worry about stressing my body?

Does any of that sound familiar to you?

It took me almost my entire pregnancy to discover all those answers. And so, once I'd gone through it myself, I was inspired to write this book for you: *The 30-Minute Pregnancy Workout Book.*

I've combined the knowledge I've acquired over my years as a personal trainer with my own experiences as a pregnant woman and a new mother to create a simple all-encompassing pregnancy book. *The 30-Minute Pregnancy Workout Book* covers more than just the nine months of pregnancy. It will help you get strong, healthy, and confident before your pregnancy, maintain fitness throughout, and show you how to get back into a shape you are comfortable with afterwards. This book provides you with a healthy way of eating and a reasonable weight lifting program you can maintain on a day-to-day basis.

We'll go over the changes in your body and with your baby month by month. That way you can understand what's happening, get prepared for what's coming, and know the adjustments you'll need to make to your diet and exercise program to get through a healthy and fit pregnancy.

Decades ago, pregnant women were told to refrain from any exercise. Nowadays we understand the benefits of moderate exercise during pregnancy, both for the unborn baby and the pregnant woman. Exercise has helped to produce healthier, happier, and more well-adjusted expectant mothers.

Even so, some pregnant women feel nervous about using free weights when doing some exercises. They think doing so will make them too bulky or overly muscular. They may reject weight lifting and bodybuilding as grotesque and unattractive. But by using free weights properly, a woman can achieve flexibility and strength in her body and a youthfulness that will serve her well over the years.

I commend you on your goal to be lean and strong, even while pregnant. You've come this far, and that is a good thing. Let's get started.

1. Before Pregnancy

The exercises featured in this chapter are:

Drop-Down Press

Jumps

Clean and Snap

Drop Press

Front Squat

Okay, first off, this book is for *everyone*. If you're one of those people who looks at magazine covers and photo spreads and thinks, *I could never be like that*, then it's meant for you in particular. Don't be put off by those pictures. Anyone can get in shape and stay in shape. It might not have been easy for you to find the motivation to be fit before now, but this is a *great* time to do it.

I'm a personal trainer and a fitness model, and I've appeared in numerous national magazines. Exercise is such a part of my everyday routine that I didn't want it to change when I discovered I was pregnant. Like most women, I'd heard stories about what pregnancy could do to your mind and body: the pregnancy weight you could never lose, the cellulite, a loss of identity, being overwhelmed by the new baby and a whole new lifestyle. I wanted to be able to keep my weight down and keep my body in roughly the same condition—for me, but also for my baby.

Actually, that brings me to a good second point—let's take a moment to talk about personal trainers. As I said, I'm one myself, and I've worked with many others. However, there have also been long stretches when I didn't have a trainer, and I worked alone. People think having a trainer is some kind of exclusive privilege, almost elitist, but in reality it's usually more of a social occasion than anything else. Sadly, many people don't want a real trainer; they just want someone to hang out with at the gym.

A trainer will not make you lose weight. He or she can help you only if you really want to do it. Money can't buy health, and some people would rather have surgery than spend an honest hour in the gym. If the motivation is coming from you, your trainer will be a guide to help you along the way. If all the motivation is coming from your trainer, you could probably be doing something more useful with your money.

Also, let me warn you: Throughout this book I'm probably going to slip a lot and refer to your baby as *she* or *her*. I'm not a psychic—I'm just very biased, going by my own experiences with my daughter, Elli.

Healthy Eating and Nutrition

Lots of people cringe at the world *diet*. It's come to have many negative connotations. Don't be scared if I mention diet over the next few pages. No one is going to suggest starving yourself or your baby. All we're talking about is *what* you eat, not how much of it you eat.

Too many people grab health bars and protein shakes instead of real meals. Have you ever read the ingredients in one of those shakes? More to the point, have you ever understood them? Don't fall victim to a corporate marketing ploy. Eat meals that have real food in them.

Eating right is one of the easiest ways to good health. A few years ago, a friend of mine decided to start seeing a personal trainer. The day after his first meeting, though, he was in a bad car crash that sprained his right arm and fractured several of his ribs. At first he was depressed, since he obviously wasn't going to be exercising, but he decided he could at least start following the new patterns of eating his trainer had set out for him. After a month of mending, doing nothing but sitting on the couch and watching television, he'd lost eight pounds.

If you want to make changes to your eating patterns, it's important to start the process before you become pregnant. Pregnancy is not a time to radically alter your diet.

Eating Meals During Pregnancy

First of all, meal portions should be frequent and small, roughly the size of the palm of your hand. While it is not a good idea to overeat, a pregnant woman should be eating enough to provide fuel to her baby. One of the worst things a pregnant woman can do is starve herself during the day and then eat one big meal at night. Protein is very important for a pregnant woman, and she should also remember to eat vegetables and carbs, and to drink plenty of water throughout the day, especially when exercising.

There's no need to exaggerate one's calorie intake and consume more than is required. It's not recommended to take in much sugar during pregnancy, because it stimulates the baby. Coffee, because of its caffeine content, is also a no-no, as are fast foods because they are high in fat and sugar. Pregnant women should allow themselves a "pig-out day" when they can indulge in having one of their favorite foods. That, however, will produce a sluggish, overworked feeling, and they are likely to want to pass up the chance to go on a food binge again.

Smart Meal Planning

How many of us have been to restaurants like the Cheesecake Factory? The meal portions are huge, easily enough for two or three people, and then you follow that up with dessert....

We have choices in everything. My favorite saying is "You are what you eat." Few people really think about what that means. Everything we eat while we are pregnant is actually what the baby is going to become. It is said that even the fat cells in your baby are determined while you are pregnant.

Stop for a second, consider what's on your plate, and ask yourself, Do I need this? Do you really need a second helping of it? Is your mind just playing tricks on you because you're depressed or need to comfort yourself? Smart eating and meal planning are essential to having a healthy baby.

The Exercises

There's a current trend in fitness that reflects our fast-paced society. People are rushing through exercises, cramming weights, cardio, and kickboxing into half an hour and then forgetting about it for the rest of the day—sometimes the rest of the week! That works fine in the short term, but years from now you'll be finding or developing injuries, and you'll have no idea where they're coming from. Why? Well, because you forgot about them.

The results of exercises should be functional—you should be able to see and experience them. If you can't be aware of your body, something needs to change. When you're pregnant, it's even more important to take the time to do things right.

The exercises in this book offer you a full-body workout in about half an hour, working whole muscle groups instead of focusing on individual body parts. When muscles are isolated and worked, your body will become imbalanced and look disproportionate. That is why you frequently meet people at the gym who have phenomenal builds but seem hunched or badly proportioned. They've developed some muscles but not others.

Here is the routine I'd been doing before discovering I was pregnant. It incorporates

Olympic-style weight lifting exercises. That may sound a bit scary at first (much like that word *diet*), but the exercises will give you that functional improvement we were just talking about. There is no single repetitious move that will put strain on your joints and ligaments. Instead, this routine will help improve your strength and flexibility.

Olympic Training

Drop-Down Press (Snatch Drop)

Jumps

Clean and Snap (Clean and Jerk)

Drop Press (Snatch Press)

Front Squat

NOTE: Snatch Drop, Clean and Jerk, and Snatch Press are the correct Olympic terms for the exercises described in the following section, but we've changed them to more commonly understood terms.

Olympic training exercises could be done by women before pregnancy, but any healthy woman can also do these exercises. There are five exercises in this chapter, but throughout the book, the equipment needed is very basic—an Olympic bar, a variety of free weights (preferably silver weights, which stay tighter to the body than rubber weights), a flat bench, and a floor mat. The recommended starting weight is five to twenty-five pounds. All the necessary equipment can be purchased at any major fitness retailer.

As we start to go through the routines, I'll explain each new exercise you will be doing.

Drop-Down Press
With a ten-pound Olympic Bar

Stand up straight with your feet hips-width apart. The bar rests on your shoulders behind your neck, with your elbows pointing down. Your hands should be wider than your shoulders, and a good way to check placement is simply to raise the bar. As you do, your arms should lock at a forty-five-degree angle.

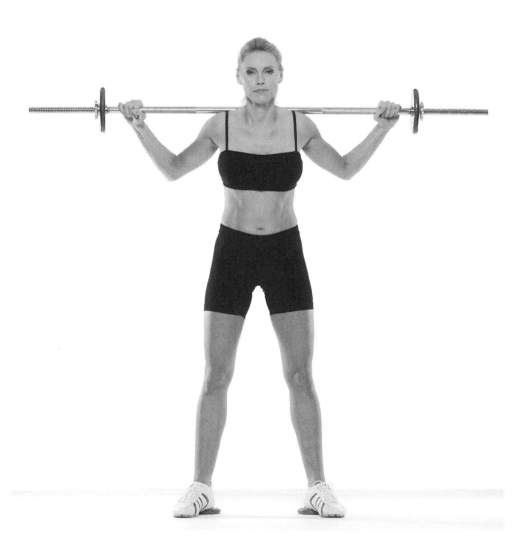

Take in a breath, and drop into a squat beneath the bar. Arch your back and keep your chin up. The object here is not to raise the bar, but to drop under it and straighten your arms, locking your elbows to hold it in place.

Now that you have the bar over you, straighten your legs and lift, exhaling as you do. All the work is being done by your legs, not your arms. Once you're standing straight, lower the bar slowly back onto your shoulders. That's one repetition.

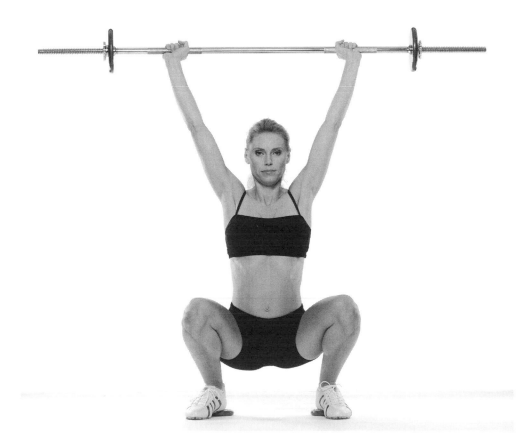

Jumps

Stand with your feet hips-width apart. The bar hangs in front of you, with your hands about shoulders-width apart. Keeping your chin up, chest out, and back arched, bend at the knees until the bar is below your knees. This is your start position.

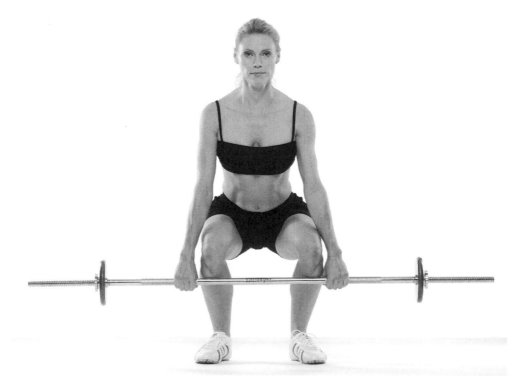

Inhale and push up hard. As the bar passes your hips, push out and give it a nudge. When your legs straighten all the way, give an extra push and make the move a little jump. You should land in the start position and exhale. That's one repetition.

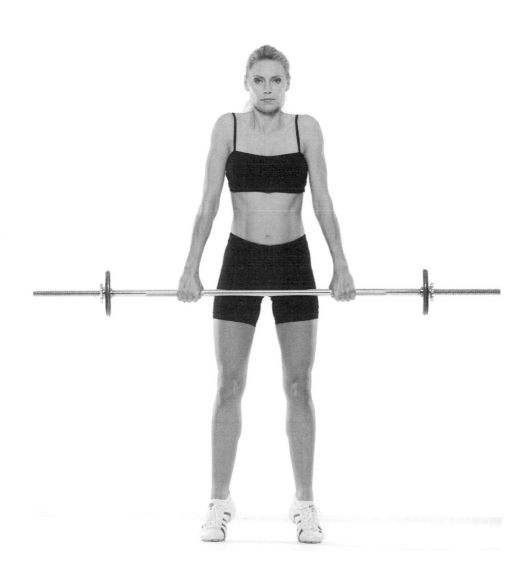

Clean and Snap

This exercise starts just like the Jump. Stand with your feet hips-width apart. The bar is on the floor in front of you. Bend at the knees, keeping your chin up, chest out, and back arched, until you can grab the bar with your hands shoulders-width apart.

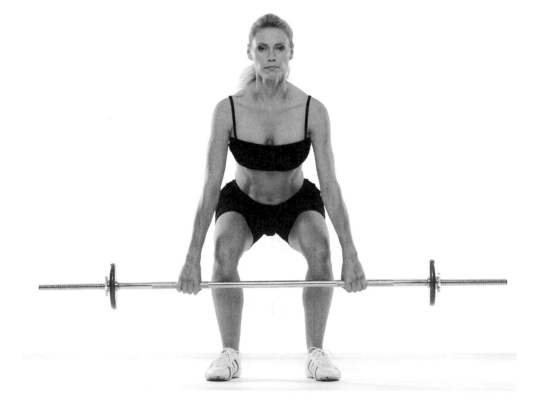

Inhale and push up hard. This time, as the bar passes your thighs, give it a little bounce and let it roll up under your chin. Don't let it swing out and throw you off balance. Keep the line of motion close to your body. End with your hands under the bar, palms up, elbows pointing out. Don't let your elbows drift down, because that can also throw you off balance.

Once you're standing straight, you can let the bar drop to the floor and exhale. That's one repetition.

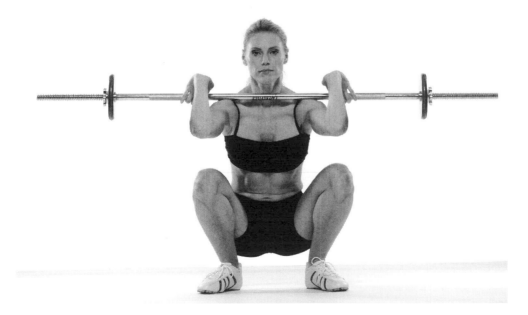

Drop Press

This can't be stressed enough: Go slow the first few times you do this exercise. I've come dangerously close to smacking myself in the chin with the bar, so until you feel comfortable, take it slow. Nothing is more embarrassing than knocking yourself out with a piece of gym equipment.

Feet are hips-width apart, and the bar is already under your chin, resting across the front of your shoulders. Palms are up, elbows are up, and your hands are shoulders-width apart.

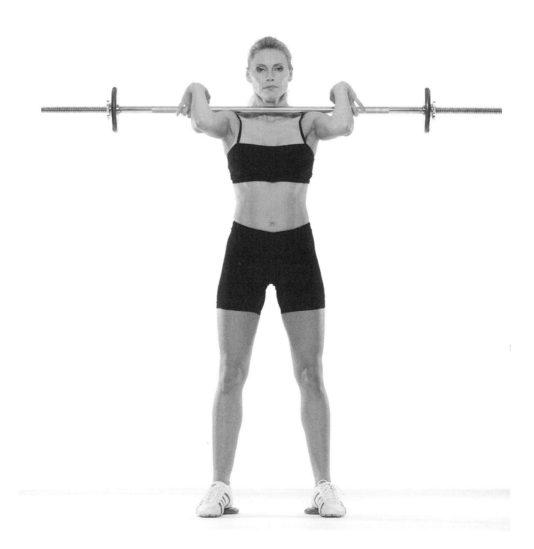

Inhale, tighten your abs, and squat. Keep your back arched, chin and elbows up.

Drop down until your knees are slightly bent and arms are locked above your shoulders. Remember, back arched, chin up, elbows up. When you return to your starting position, lower the bar slowly back to your shoulders, keeping your knees soft and slightly bent. This prevents too much weight being borne by the knees. When you're standing straight again, that's one repetition.

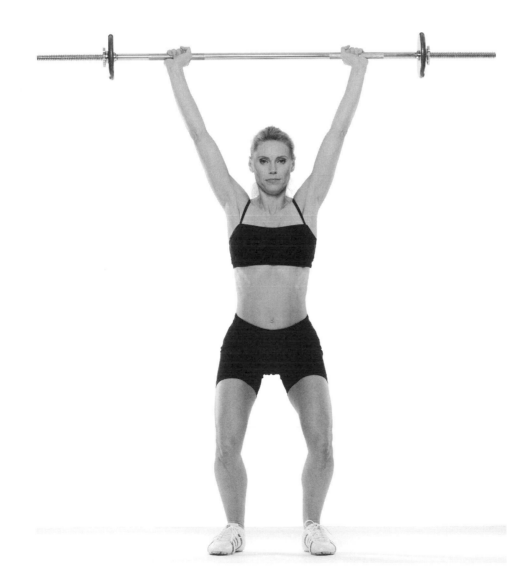

Front Squat

Stand with your feet hips-width apart. Hold the weight in front of you with both hands, keeping your elbows as high as you can. That will help stop you from leaning forward with your squat.

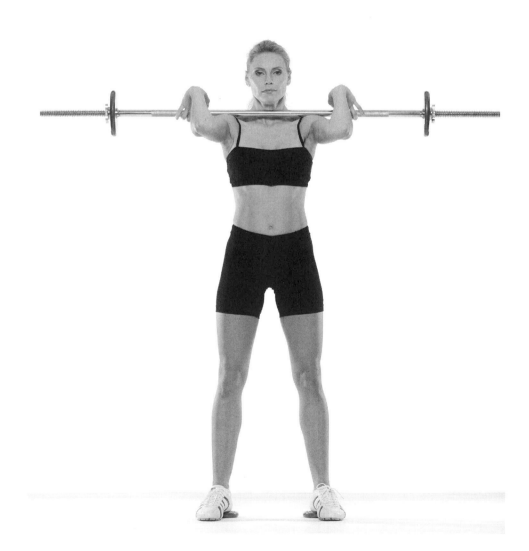

Inhale, drop your body under the bar, and straighten your arms. This won't be a big drop, since the bar is starting fairly high, so you shouldn't end up in a deep crouch. Keep your back arched the whole time to maintain your balance. Once your arms lock, push your legs straight, raising the bar. Once your knees are straight, exhale and lower the bar back to your shoulders. When the bar lands across your shoulders, let your knees bend to help absorb the weight. That's one repetition.

If you don't have the flexibility to perform this exercise, put a board or a rolled-up towel under your heels (and only your heels), so your feet are tilted forward slightly. This will give you a little lift and should make the exercise easier.

Remember, go slow at first.

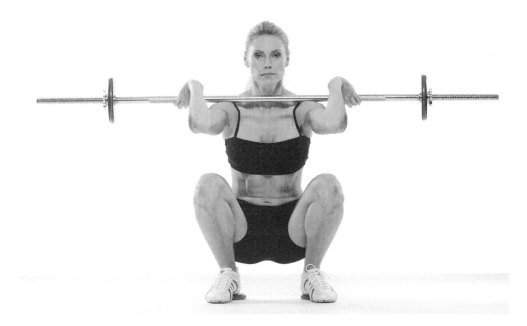

The exercises should be performed three times a week straight through as outlined in the order presented in the book. It is better to work the body as a whole rather than to exhaust the smaller muscle groups in your upper body. It's not a good idea to isolate the exercises for different body parts, meaning you shouldn't do exercises for arms one day, then do leg exercises another day.

Doing the exercises three times a week is ideal, but if not, once a week is better than nothing at all. The weight levels used largely depend on the fitness and health of the person. And remember, the weight range is only recommended levels.

Weight levels increase and decrease depending on the exercises performed. When doing upper-body exercises, it's generally accepted that small weights (five to twenty-five pounds) be used, for lower-body exercises use bigger weights (ten to forty-five pounds). The upper body is weaker than the much stronger and firmer legs and torso, so small weights are needed when doing these exercises. Of course, as a person becomes more flexible and their fitness level increases, larger weights can be used on an upper-body exercise routine.

Back in the Exercise Game

If you did the Olympic training program prior to becoming pregnant you should wait at least four to six weeks after giving birth before starting any kind of exercise program. The length of time before starting to exercise also depends on whether you had a C-section or natural childbirth. If you had a C-section, it's not advisable to start with the Olympic training program right away, but start with the Time Trials (outlined in chapter 2) as a way to rebuild your body first. Then, in about two months, you can begin to incorporate the Olympic training program and alternate it with Time Trials.

A Few More Notes

You're starting now, and that's good. You've begun to make positive choices for yourself that are going to reflect on that baby you're thinking about having, even if you're not planning to have a baby right away.

Try not to worry about those changes. Lots of people think changing their eating habits will have a huge impact on their social life, and on their life in general. Make up a simple and smart meal plan that you can stick to and live with it. The same holds for the exercises. They shouldn't be a chore, or something you *have* to do. Make them something you *want* to do.

And now that you've made these choices, let's move on to the next big step, probably the reason you picked up this book.

2. The First Trimester

The exercises featured in this chapter are:

Hammer

Triceps Extension

Crunches

Dead Lift

Standing Fly

Standing Row

Stiff Leg Dead Lift

Crunches (straight leg)

Reverse Hammer

Side Crunches

Pullover

Front Squat

P art of my regular exercise routine was neuromuscular massage. It's a deep, hard, cleansing form of massage that helps rid the body of toxins. My massage therapist, Barrance, had been doing this work for years and was a consummate professional.

Since my previous session, though, I'd been sick with an upset stomach and I had thrown up almost every morning. Barrance had worked on my stomach quite a bit that last time, and I wondered if he had done something wrong. I called him, and he reassured me that nothing he'd done was causing my symptoms.

"You probably just have the flu, a mild case of food poisoning, or something," he said. Then he chuckled and added, "Hey, maybe you're pregnant." We had a good laugh and hung up.

After another week of nausea, though, I started to wonder....Maybe it wouldn't hurt to check. I bought a home pregnancy test, used it the next morning, and was shocked when it gave me an immediate positive result. I scheduled an appointment with my gynecologist, and it was confirmed: I was eight weeks pregnant.

"Congratulations," Dr. Katz said. "I guess we'll be seeing you again."

My situation wasn't unique. Many pregnancies are unplanned, and many women don't discover they are pregnant until well into their first trimester. There is very little weight gain, so it's easy to make my mistake and write off other symptoms to this or that.

Morning sickness is the classic first sign of pregnancy. It strikes only some women, and even then some worse than others. As I said, I was one of the lucky ones.

No one knows exactly what causes the queasiness and vomiting, although rising levels of hormones are a prime suspect, especially human chorionic gonadotropin (HCG), a hormone produced by the placenta that maintains the corpeus luteum during pregnancy. It can occur at any time of the day, even all day long.

If you suffer from morning sickness, you may not feel like eating, but it's even more important that you do eat. An intake of complex carbohydrates can help decrease your nausea. Eating smaller, more frequent meals will also help because acid production increases in an empty stomach. Drinking fluids may make you feel worse, but preventing dehydration is vitally important, especially if you are vomiting.

There are, as you're aware of by now, dozens of home remedies for morning sickness. Peppermint tea in various forms, ginger, and crackers also help. Remember, never take motion sickness pills or nausea medications without first speaking to your doctor.

When you realize you're pregnant, however it happens, you're also going to need a series of tests done. Most of them will be done right there in your doctor's office, just as they confirm your pregnancy. Some need to be sent to laboratories for full results. My tests were so overwhelming at the time, I honestly don't remember half of them, but these are the ones you should expect:

Once the pregnancy has been confirmed, an initial blood test is done to screen for anemia, hepatitis B, rubella, chicken pox, and also to determine your blood type and Rh status.

The Rh factor is a protein found in the red blood cells of some people. (That is why you hear of blood being positive or negative—it depends on whether you have the protein or not.) If you are Rh-negative and your fetus is Rh-positive, your body may possibly attack the baby's red blood cells, seeing them as an infection. If an Rh difference is detected, the doctor will provide shots to prevent such an immune system reaction.

Your blood pressure will be taken at your first appointment and at every checkup. In the case of an abnormally high or low blood pressure, you will need to be closely monitored.

There will also be a urine check to confirm the appropriate protein and sugar levels and to detect any urinary tract infections. If you haven't had one on a usual visit, a Pap smear is also necessary to check for cancerous cells in your cervix.

The first visit will also include a variety of tests for AIDS and other STIs. If untreated, these infections can cause birth defects and pregnancy complications. A glucose screening can help assess the risk of gestational diabetes, which can result in overly large babies, difficult deliveries, and birth trauma. You'll drink a sweet glucose drink, and an hour later a blood sample is drawn from your arm and sent to a lab for testing.

A sample of chorionic villi (the tiny fingerlike tissues of placenta) is obtained in either of two ways: through a tube inserted in the vagina and cervix, or by means of a needle guided into the abdomen with the help of ultrasound. The sample is then tested in a lab to detect chromosomal disorders such as Down syndrome and also some genetic disorders such as sickle-cell anemia, cystic fibrosis, and Tay-Sachs disease.

Amniocentesis can detect a number of genetic and chromosomal disorders and also confirm the baby's sex. A long needle is guided through the abdomen with the help of ultrasound. The small sample of amniotic fluid that is removed gets tested in a lab.

Even though it's a bit scary, we should talk a bit about miscarriages. There are many reasons women miscarry. Often a fetus's chromosomes are damaged, or it could have too few of them or too many, and that may result in a miscarriage. Most pregnancies proceed normally, but can develop certain complications later on.

One rare but life-threatening complication (for you and the embryo) is ectopic pregnancy, in which the fertilized egg implants outside the uterus, in the abdomen or in a fallopian tube. Symptoms include sudden intense pain in the lower abdomen. If not treated by surgical means, ectopic pregnancy can result in massive internal bleeding and even death.

Your doctor should also screen your family health history for possible genetic problems. You should discuss any medications you may be using to make sure they won't be harmful to a growing fetus.

What You and Your Baby Are Doing

One thing to remember as we go over these facts is that every pregnancy is different. Your baby may gain weight faster, or start kicking earlier. There are no hard, solid rules. That's why I've tried not to pin too many things to specific weeks, so you get more of a general feel of where your baby is in his or her development.

Doctors date a pregnancy beginning with the first day of your last period, which is called the gestation age method. Most people don't realize they're pregnant until their fourth week or so. Sometimes you might not even know until week eight, like me.

Many women feel increased sexual desire at the time of ovulation, which occurs fourteen days before the next period comes. To accurately predict it, you can use an ovulation detection kit. In couples with normal fertility, the frequency with which you have sex isn't important so long as the sperm are there in time to meet up with the egg.

It all begins when the sperm contacts the outer surface of the egg, eventually fusing with it. Without activation from sperm, an egg typically remains dormant and soon dies. It's fertilization that sets the egg on an irreversible pathway of cell division and embryo development. After fusion, the fertilized egg is called a zygote, and once the zygote divides to a two-cell stage, it's called an embryo or, more specifically, a blastocyst.

Within a few hours of fertilization, your baby's sex, eye color, and hair texture have already been set. Your fertilized egg will divide into identical cells as it travels through the fallopian tube and into the uterus. The uterus has already formed a lush bed of tissues, and the blastocyst embeds itself in that wall. Implantation triggers the production of HCG, the hormone that turns your pregnancy test positive and may cause morning sickness. I've mentioned human chorionic gonadotropin before, and here's where it comes from.

There aren't any visible signs of pregnancy right now, but your body is undergoing profound changes, leaving you exhausted. Fatigue and mood swings may set in, making it very difficult to find energy and motivation for your exercise. Exercise in general will work wonders in keeping your energy levels up. If you need a special diet to manage allergies, diabetes, or maternal obesity, see a registered dietitian. Your breasts may be starting to get hard and sore. You may still have all the usual PMS symptoms.

After the first few weeks, the blastocyst has developed a few primitive organs and rough arms, legs, eyes, and ears. There is a distinct heart, though, quite an accomplishment when you realize that he or she is barely one-sixteenth of an inch long (about the thickness of a quarter).

The placenta and the umbilical cord are fully functioning by week five, passing oxygen and nutrients between you and the embryo, which is now almost the size of a pea. You are officially hooked up to your baby now. The fluid-filled amniotic sac has formed, and other major organs are developing.

The embryo is taking a more human shape, and bone starts to replace cartilage. There are ears, a nose, and stubby little webbed fingers and toes. The eyes are well developed, but for now they're covered by a membrane lid and still more on the side of the head than at the front.

Your cervix is tightly closed now, and your uterus is slowly enlarging while your waistline expands a bit. You're going to start bloating, partly because of pregnancy hormones, partly because your digestive organs are functioning slower than usual. You may notice certain changes, such as your facial skin becoming smoother, or there may be an outbreak of pimples. Your breasts may be fuller or slightly tender.

By the start of the third month, your morning sickness should be letting up, but your hair, nails, skin, and breasts may be taking on a new life of their own. A grapefruit-size uterus is probably pushing itself to the front of your abdomen.

Your abdomen may begin to pick up the fetus's rapid heartbeat on a Doppler stethoscope, recording the baby's heart rate in response to its own movement. (This is called a nonstress test.) He or she may even be moving around a little bit, although the child is probably far too tiny for you to feel it. Bones are forming, fingers are developing more, toenails are growing, and tiny buds are sprouting in her gums. (These will become teeth.) Although the sex was decided weeks ago, it's still difficult to distinguish. Your baby's eyelids meet and won't open again for nearly four months.

At the end of this first trimester, your fetus is probably about three inches long and weighs about an ounce. The heart is beating, kidneys are secreting urine, and the liver and pancreas are working. The respiratory system is working; bile and the reproductive organs, bone cells, fingers, and toes are forming. The risk of miscarriage has dropped significantly at this point.

Now let's talk more about you.

Healthy Eating and Nutrition

You're going to need an extra three hundred calories a day, but there's no need to worry about measuring and weighing everything you eat down to the last gram. Eating a well-balanced and healthy diet during pregnancy helps to maintain your own health and to nourish your baby.

The recommended weight gain during pregnancy is twenty to thirty pounds. Your weight gain may vary depending on a number of things: your age, your fitness level, what your weight was before you became pregnant, as well as the type of lifestyle you lead. Regardless, yours should be a *steady* weight gain, which comes from eating healthful foods.

Don't be selfish and think of this as your big chance to pig out on whatever you want. "Eating for two" isn't a license to go crazy. Think of your baby's health, because he or she is going to be depending on you for the next nine months. Obesity in pregnancy increases your risk of heart disease, diabetes, and fetal distress.

At this point, we need to stop and talk about proper nutrition and how vital it is for human growth, maintenance, repair, energy, and physical performance. One of the basic rules during pregnancy is cutting down on bad fats, sugars, and caffeine. Junk food, coffee, and empty calories will not feed your baby's development, only your own fat cells.

Another reason many of us turn to food is to cope with anxiety. It's easy to feel insecure and get scared. Your daily routine is about to be changed, and nobody likes change, especially such a drastic one. Sugar can make you feel good because it increases the amount of a brain chemical called serotonin. Serotonin is a neurotransmitter, and it makes you feel satisfied and relaxed after eating. Vegetables and whole grains can also increase serotonin production, but the effect does not set in so immediately. Don't go for the quick fix.

During pregnancy, you may begin to experience strange cravings. Try to avoid sweets when you crave them. Eating artificial sugars can actually increase morning sickness, and it puts your blood sugar level on a roller-coaster ride. Before you eat, think about whether the food you crave is going to satisfy your baby's needs or just your own appetite.

Behavior counts as much as biology, and the primary reason we get hooked on junk food is because of the misguided intentions of our parents. Okay, sermon's over. Back to the baby.

Proper nutrition is important to fetal development. Most organs and structures develop within the first two months of pregnancy. Think about it: A human body is being built from the ground up. All the nutrients you use to maintain your body are needed as raw materials for that new baby. When you don't get enough protein, your muscles feel weak, but that fetus is trying to *create* muscles.

On that note, protein is the most important caloric nutrient for your baby. More than half your (and her) dry body mass is made up of protein—large, heavy molecules composed of amino acids. There are about twenty different amino acids, eight of which are essential to your good health. Your body uses those amino acids to build new proteins, which in turn are used to build new cells (for you and especially for baby) and maintain old ones. Protein is also a source of energy for your body.

Unrefined, high-fiber carbohydrates will give you sustained energy. They can also reduce morning sickness, indigestion, and constipation. A high complex-carbohydrate intake is very important, and in the first and second trimester, those carbohydrates play a big part in the development of the fetus.

Fat is our energy storage. In the first trimester, your body will deposit little fat pillows to protect the pregnancy. Some fat is essential, but only a small amount is needed to meet basic nutritional needs. Honest.

Water lubricates joints; fills muscles, tissues, organs, blood; and helps to maintain your body temperature. When you're pregnant, you need to avoid dehydration, which will slow blood and nutrient flow to your baby and increase your body temperature.

Your doctor will prescribe some prenatal vitamins. Remember that many vitamins and minerals have a degree of toxicity that could be dangerous to you and your baby if you start overdosing on them. Be very careful with any nonprescribed vitamin and mineral supplements.

Vitamin A is important for the growth and repair of many tissues in your body, and it aids in the development of bones and teeth. It's also important for developing strong eyes. Since your baby is building a body from scratch, he or she will definitely need vitamin A.

Your body uses vitamin B6 to help metabolize proteins, fats, and carbs. You're taking in more of all of these, so you'll probably need a little more B6, too. As an added plus, it can help with morning sickness.

Vitamin B1 (sometimes called thiamin) also helps metabolize carbs, turning food into energy. Your brain, nerves, and heart (and your baby) all need B1 to work properly. It also helps with growth and muscle development.

It's very easy to lose potassium, especially if you're prone to morning sickness, as I was. Bananas are a great way to get it back. Potassium helps to keep your body's fluids in balance, and to make your kidneys filter and eliminate toxins.

And you've heard it before, but I'll say it again: Stay away from alcohol, cigarettes, and drugs!

The Exercises

So, here we are. This is why you bought the book. First things first—you've heard this before, but check with your doctor before you begin. Your doctor knows you better than I do, and will have a better idea of what you're capable of. If you don't like what you hear, get a second opinion. You know yourself better than anyone else, but if every doctor and medical professional you consult is saying exercise isn't for you, you might want to consider their advice.

No matter what, though, you need to remember that you are carrying a baby now, and nothing in this book is going to help you lift more than you could before you were pregnant. If you weren't very active prepregnancy, ease into these exercises.

There were two things Dr. Katz recommended to me, and you should know both of them. First, drink lots of fluids. You're prone to dehydration right now, and it can sneak up on you much faster than you'd think. As we've just detailed, dehydration can be deadly to your baby, so take a bottle of water to the gym and drink all of it, even if you're not feeling thirsty.

Second, your new best friend will be a heart rate monitor. Your heart rate should never go over 140 beats per minute. For the next nine months, putting extra pressure on your system means putting extra pressure on your baby's system, which is extremely delicate. You can pick up a heart rate monitor for between thirty and two hundred dollars.

If you're already working out on a regular basis, you don't need to change your routine that much. In fact, you really don't need to follow this trimester's workout if you don't want to. You probably want to cut your weights down by about half, just to reduce some of the strain and to ease your heart rate a bit. The first trimester is going to be easy for you.

If this book is your first real attempt at exercise, or if you just want to check out my plan, we're going to try something called a time trial. This is different from most exercise plans out there right now, in that it's a cardiovascular workout done with weights and weight lifting exercises. To be honest, I was doing the previous workout pretty much all through this trimester. Keep in mind, I was just shy of two months pregnant before finding out. So, looking back on things, if I'd known from day one, my workout would have been something more like this:

Time Trial

FIRST GROUP

Hammer	3 to 8 pounds
Triceps Extension	8 to 12 pounds
Crunches	
Dead Lift	10 pounds

SECOND GROUP

Standing Fly	3 to 5 pounds
Standing Row	5 to 10 pounds
Stiff-Leg Dead Lift	5 to 10 pounds
Crunches (straight leg)	

THIRD GROUP

Reverse Hammer	3 to 8 pounds
Side Crunches	
Pullover	5 to 10 pounds
Front Squat	10 pounds

You're going to do three sets of each of these exercises, doing twenty repetitions in each set. Work on each group one at a time. In other words, do all the sets of all your first-group exercises, cycling through the first group three times, before moving on to the second group.

As far as weights go, experienced people should cut their weights in half. For the rest of you, if you've been doing this only since you picked up this book, start with the recommendations above, aiming at the lower end. If it still feels easy after a week, try going up a pound or two.

First, go easy to get true flexibility and the right form going. As you are more confident, move up a pound. Remember, it's not about how much weight you are working with; these exercises are designed to be functional.

Hammer

deltoids, triceps, teres minor, biceps, pectorals, and infraspinati (muscle groups worked in the exercises)

The weight to be used depends on your fitness level. I'd recommend 3 pounds for beginners, 8 pounds for someone more advanced. Start with arms at your sides, holding the weights with your palms in, and your feet hips-width apart. Keep your chest out and your chin up. Inhale, tighten your abdominals, and lift the weights to your shoulders, straight up to the ceiling. Keep the weights close to your body the whole time. Don't swing them out in front. While pressing up, pull down with your chest; this movement will help to isolate the muscles.

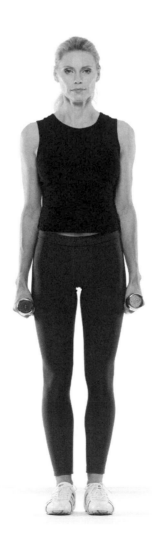

Let the weights drop back to the start position, exhaling as you do so. You've just completed one repetition. Remember to keep your spine straight and to keep the weights with your palms facing each other through the whole exercise, so they look like hammers.

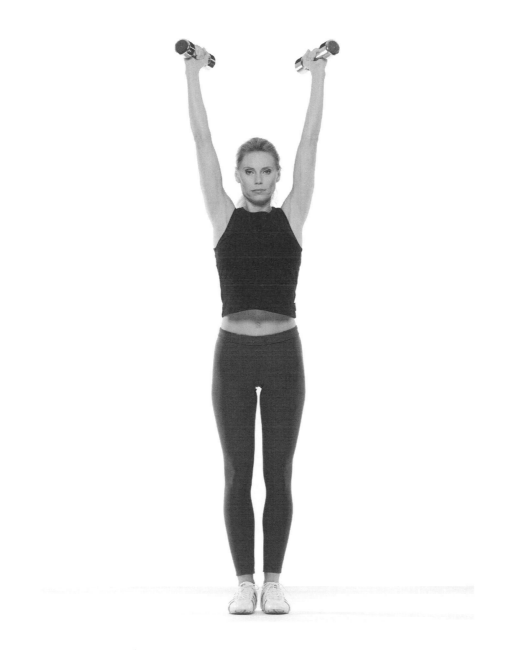

Triceps Extension
triceps, latissimi dorsi

This is one of my favorites, because it deals with a worry area. It's great for tightening up that little sag that develops under your arms.

Stand with your feet hips-width and your back straight, chest out, and chin up. Take the dumbbell in both hands behind your head, cradling one end between them. It should be hanging vertical, not held, with your elbows in tight against your head.

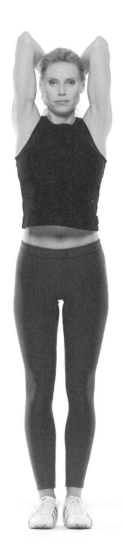

Take a first breath; then lift the weight straight behind your head, inhaling as you press up. Keep your elbows in; don't let them drift out. Exhale as you lower the weight back behind your head. That's one repetition.

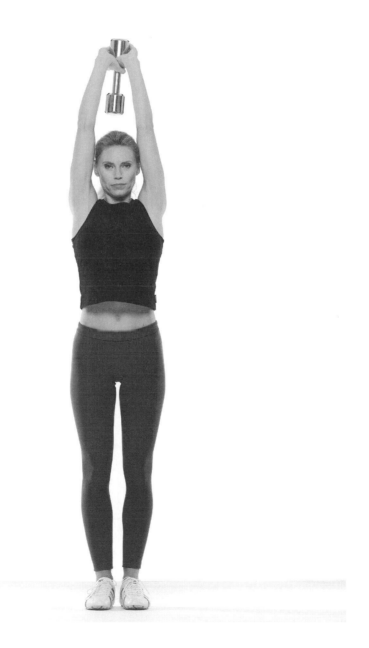

Crunches
abdominals, external obliques

Crunches are a classic exercise and great for your abs. Lie on your back on the floor mat. Make sure you push your back toward the floor. Don't arch your back or pull your head up. Lift your legs into a "sitting" position, and keep them there. You can put your hands under your head for support, but resist the urge to pull on it and strain your neck and shoulders! The only muscles you should tense for this are your abdominals.

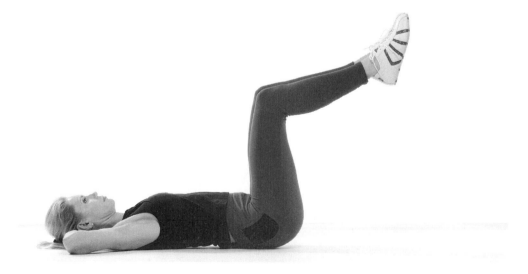

Lift your torso toward your knees. Remember, use "only" your abdominals. You're not trying to touch your knees, you're just rolling your body up and forward until all your abdominals have fired.

If you feel tension in your arms, neck, or shoulders, you need to relax them. If you're having trouble isolating your abs, do your crunches with your hands on your stomach. It's an easy way to feel when the right muscles are firing.

Once all your abdominals have clenched, relax back down until you're at the start position. That's one repetition.

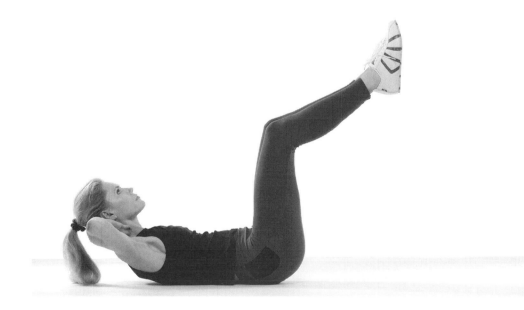

Dead Lift

will increase strength in the buttocks, lower back, spine, and groin

Stand with your feet hips-width apart, hold the weights on each side of your body, keep your chest up, and inhale. Hold your abs tight but continue to keep your chest up while bringing the weights below your knee level. Make sure you don't lean forward. Your body weight should be in the back, almost as if you're in a sitting position.

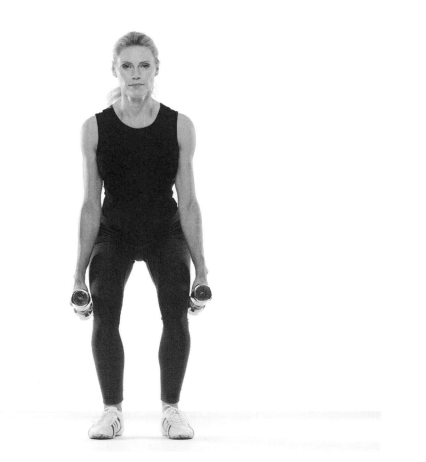

When coming back up, push yourself up from your heels and exhale. That's one repetition.

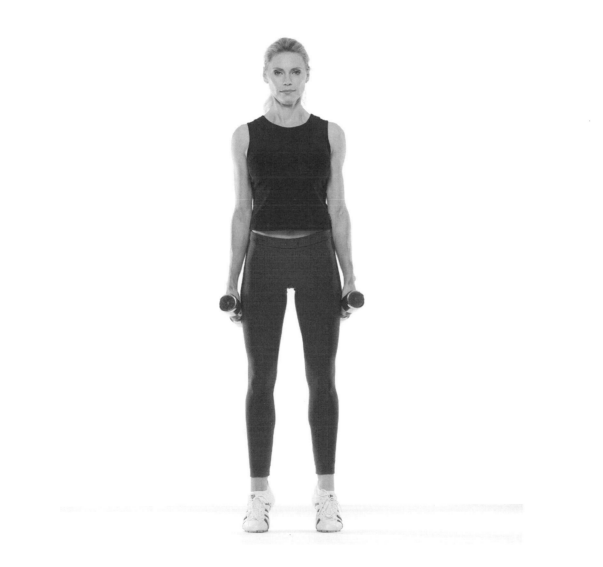

Standing Fly

deltoids, lats, teres minor, infraspinati, brachioradiales

Start with arms at your sides, weights held with your palms in, and feet together. Keep your chest out and your chin up.

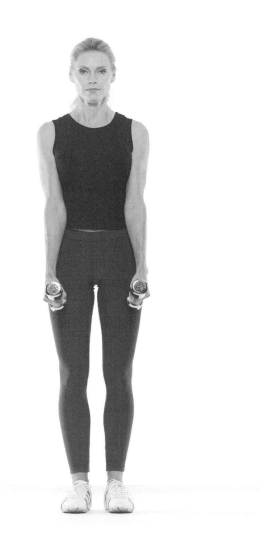

Exhale, tighten your abs, and lift your arms straight out slowly, elbows locked out to either side. Don't swing them. Keep your arms locked, and raise them to shoulder height (no higher), with your palms down.

Once you've reached your high point, exhale and lower your arms to your sides. That's one repetition.

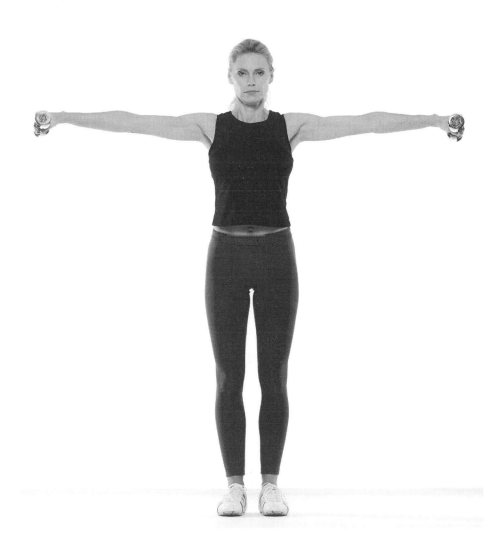

Standing Row

biceps, deltoids, triceps, lats, teres minor, infraspinati

This is an easy one, and it goes quick. (But that doesn't mean you rush through it.) Start with feet together, chest out, and chin up. Arms should be straight out in front of you, just past your thighs, with your palms in.

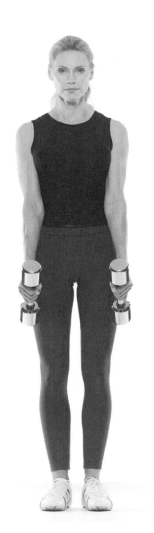

Inhaling, pull the weights up and back so they end up between your hips and your waist. Don't go higher than your waist. It's important to keep your arms moving in a straight line, so don't let your elbows drift—they should stay close to your body. Lower the weights, exhaling as you go. That's one repetition.

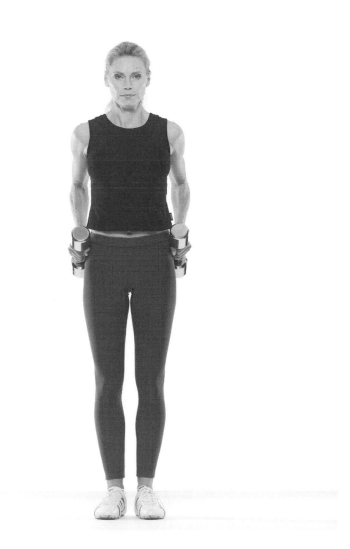

Stiff-Leg Dead Lift

glutei maximi, adductor magnus, semitendinosus solei, gastrocne-mii, Achilles tendons

Start with feet together, chest out, chin up. The weights should hang straight below your shoulders for this entire exercise.

Inhale, and bend from your hips. Your feet need to stay flat on the ground, legs straight, and your head needs to stay in line with your spine. As you go down, the weights should hang forward, always below your shoulders. Go down until your back is parallel with the floor.

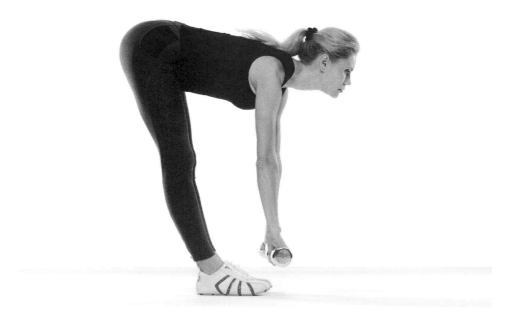

The most important part of this exercise is your back. Your back needs to stay straight and flat through this entire exercise. I can't stress this enough. If you bend your back during this movement, you're straining it. This exercise is for your butt, and if you're doing it right, that's where you'll feel it. If you can't go down all the way without bending your back, then stop just before your back goes out of line. This exercise will build your flexibility up over time, honest.

Once you've reached your low point, come back up, exhaling as you do. Push with your butt, not your toes, and keep your head in line with your back. Come up onto your toes to finish. That's one repetition.

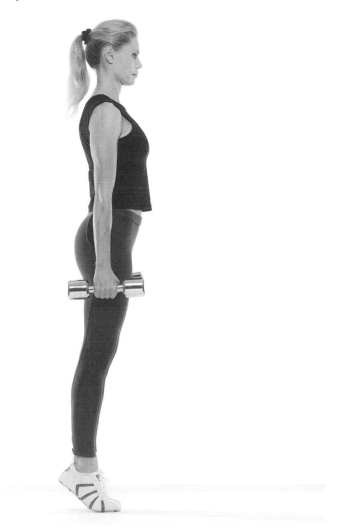

Crunches (straight leg)
to increase the flexibility of the abdomen and lower back

Lie on your back, relax the rib cage, and let your elbows lie comfortably on the floor.
Keep your neck and arms relaxed during this movement.

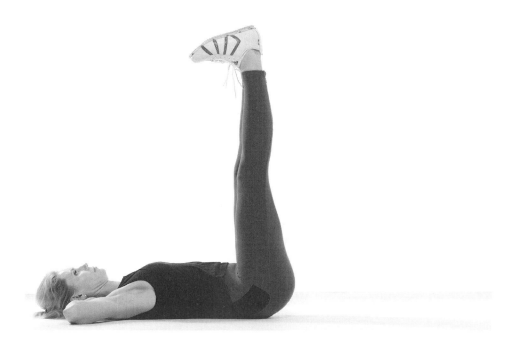

THE 30-MINUTE PREGNANCY WORKOUT BOOK

Make a conscious effort to begin lifting by firming only the abdominal muscles. Roll the upper body forward until the lower abdominal flattens. Exhale and repeat.

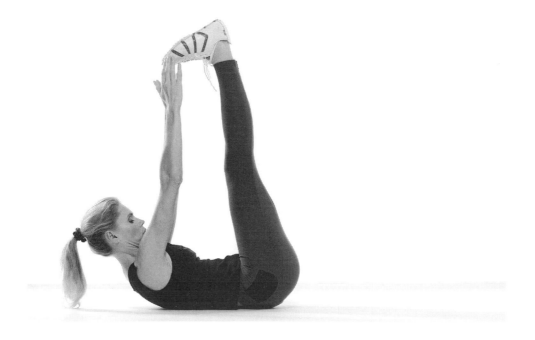

Reverse Hammer

deltoids, triceps, teres minor, biceps, pectorals, infraspinati

This exercise is almost exactly like the basic Hammer from the first group. We're just going to make one alteration to work a different part of the muscle group in your shoulders.

Start with arms at your sides, holding the weights with your palms in, and your feet together. Keep your chest out and your chin up.

Inhale, tighten your abdominals, and fire the weights to your shoulders. Turn your wrists so your shoulders and palms are now turned out and the dumbbells are now side to side. As with the basic Hammer, don't swing them.

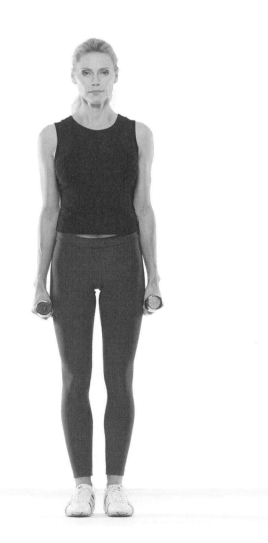

Keeping your abs tight, exhale and press the weights up until your arms are straight. While pressing up, pull down with your chest; this will help isolate the muscles.

Let the weights drop back to the start position, palms back in, inhaling as you do. You've just completed one repetition.

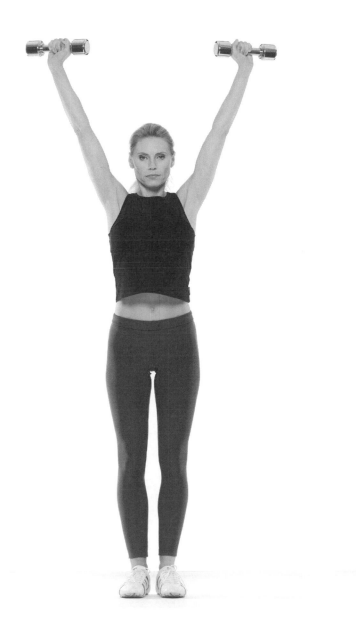

Side Crunches
to increase your strength in the obliques side by the abdominal muscles that support the spine

Lie on the floor with your legs straight, press your back onto the floor, rest your head in your hands—but don't pull on your head. Inhale, bring your right knee into your chest and, at the same time, raise your left shoulder blade from the floor in the direction of your knee and exhale.

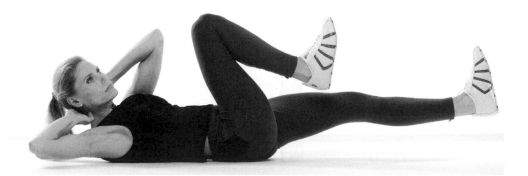

Return your right leg and left shoulder to the starting position, inhale, bring your left knee into your chest, and meet it with your right elbow, alternate the sides, and exhale.

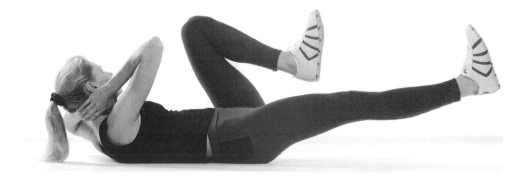

Pullover
lats, teres minor, infraspinati, pecs, abdominals

Lie down on your mat, holding one weight in both hands directly above your chest. Keep your abs tight and your back flat against the mat. You don't want your back to arch during this exercise. Inhaling as you go, lower the weight back until your arms are straight "over" your head. Lock your arms as you move, or you'll be working (and straining) the wrong muscles.

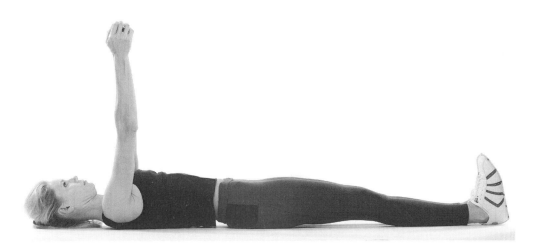

Now, keeping your arms straight and exhaling, lift the weight over your head and back to the start position. That's one repetition.

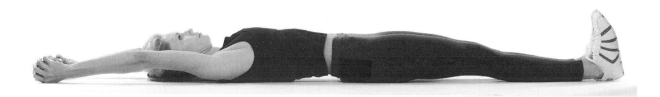

Front Squat

(with free weight) to increase the strength and flexibility in the quadriceps and buttocks, and to improve your posture by strengthening the lower back and abs

Stand upright with your feet hips-width apart. Hold the weight in front of you with both hands, keeping your elbows as high as you can. This will help stop you from leaning forward with your squat.

Inhale, tighten your abs, and squat. Keep your back straight, chin and elbows up. Go down until you're sitting on your calves. Go as far as you can while keeping your back straight.

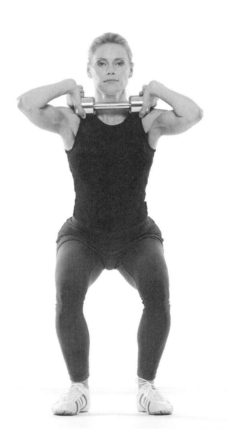

Push yourself back up, exhaling, making your buttocks work. (Come up on your toes.) Remember: back straight, chin up, elbows up. When you're standing straight again, that's one repetition.

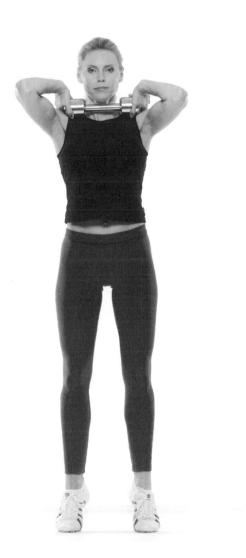

Ten Fitness Tips

1. NO GUILT. If the workout becomes too strenuous, take a guilt-free day off to recharge your batteries for the next day.

2. THE SPA LIFE. A day at the spa with a massage, bath, and other pampering is a good way to reward yourself.

3. DRINK UP. Exercising can be intense, so it's important to drink plenty of water to replace those lost fluids.

4. DARK AND TASTY. Everybody loves dark chocolate, and it's good for you. Have a chocolate snack when you get the urge, but only in moderation.

5. THE BUDDY SYSTEM. Make your fitness routine fun and enjoyable. For example, go with your partner, friend, or a neighbor to a yoga class.

6. WALK IT OFF. A simple brisk walk around the block is an excellent exercise to relieve stress at home.

7. AT THE MOVIES. Join a movie club where pregnant women and new mothers go with their babies to watch family-friendly matinee films.

8. BODY HEAT. Your body temperature rises during a workout, so make sure the exercise room is a cool (not cold) environment.

9. LET'S MAMBO. Choose your favorite piece of music to play during your exercise routine; it makes the experience more enjoyable.

10. SAFETY FIRST. Think on your feet when doing exercises. Don't overexert yourself—there's always tomorrow.

A Few More Notes

This first trimester is when everything can overwhelm you. Your whole routine is about to change, and it's easy to get insecure when it feels as if whole sections of your life are being shut down or put on hold. This is that fear of change we talked about earlier. Changes in your lifestyle, in your shape, inside your own body. It's easy to let food become a comfort for you, and from there it's easy to get lazy, too.

Don't let your insecurity get that far. Talk with your spouse, your family, and your friends. Let your loved ones know what you're feeling and what you're thinking. One of the worst things you can do for insecurities is bottle them up and let them grow.

Exercising will help keep your energy and your confidence up. You'll be able to go through this pregnancy with a great attitude, and it all starts right here.

Don't forget that heart monitor.

3. The Second Trimester

The exercises featured in this chapter are:

Flys

Rear Shoulder

Side Bends

Squat on Bench

Bench Pullover

Standing Row

Twist

Dead Lift

Bicep Curls with a Twist

Kickback

Leg Lifts

Stiff-Leg Dead Lift

was getting a lot of satisfaction being a personal trainer in Los Angeles and soon stopped modeling and acting due to my commitment to learn everything about the fitness world. All that changed when I got pregnant. Despite the fact that I was still slim and still exercising, people were starting to see me as a frail thing who needed to take things easy and be looked after. Some of my clients began to cancel appointments.

What felt even worse, though, were the ones that I needed to cancel. The truth was, I did have to cut back a bit, and there were some exercises I couldn't do. What kind of trainer works with people when she can't help them or guide them? So, I had to tell a few of my clients that we wouldn't be able to work together again until after the baby was born.

On the plus side, the free time was letting me hone this workout and gather all the information I'm now sharing with you.

One of the best things about this trimester is pictures. You can start a big collection of baby pictures right now.

An ultrasound is used to check the expected due date, to monitor high-risk pregnancies, and also to check the position of the fetus and placenta. Later in the pregnancy, when the genitals are visible, the baby's sex can also be confirmed with an ultrasound.

Also, it costs a little more, but the next step up is a 4-D ultrasound. It provides incredibly clear pictures of your baby moving in the womb. The traditional 2-D scan you have at twenty weeks is a fuzzy image, and only a trained eye can pick out the baby's features. The 4-D scanner enables doctors to pick up any abnormalities earlier and more accurately. It lets them study the surface anatomy of the baby, and you can see it smile, frown, or yawn. It's an excellent device for studying the baby's movements.

You also may want to start taking naps during the day, unless it makes you sleepless at night. Put your feet up and rest as often as you can during the day. In order to sleep comfortably at night, you might find it helpful to place a pillow under your belly for support and a pillow between your knees, as well. As your pregnancy advances, don't sleep on your back. It's safer to lie on your left side. That way the large blood vessel in front of your backbone won't be blocked by the increasing weight of your uterus.

What You and Your Baby Are Doing

As the second trimester begins, around week thirteen, your fetus looks more and more like a tiny human being. This is a phase of rapid growth, when your baby is going to be developing in jumps and bursts. The legs start to lengthen and get more proportional to the arms. Her permanent thin skin is entirely covered with an ultrafine layer of hair called lanugo. The heartbeat is getting stronger, and the baby is probably performing simple functions like sleeping, waking, kicking, swallowing, even urinating.

By the end of the fourth month, the fetus is now nourished by the placenta and probably weighs almost eight ounces (half a pound). You've probably started to feel some movement. It's actually not unusual for the baby to start sucking his or her thumb right around now.

From here on, you might be putting on half a pound per week, perhaps as much as a full pound if you're not so active. And food never tasted so good. You are full of energy and might feel sexier at times. You should enjoy your workouts much more now.

As your uterus is growing bigger and heavier, it will put more pressure on the vena cava (the vein that returns blood from your legs to the heart). It's best to avoid lying on your back. Doing so makes you dizzy and decreases the flow of oxygen to your baby. Your heart is beating faster because it has to work harder. Because of that, you cannot rely on the old heart rate to monitor your workout intensity any longer.

By the middle of this trimester, as this rapid-growth phase comes to an end, your baby is becoming more developed. The cheeks and bridge of the nose have appeared, and the eyes come closer together on the front of the skull. Eyelids and eyebrows have probably formed by the twentieth week or so, and the bones of the inner ear have hardened and taken on more definition. He or she has almost doubled in mass at this point, weighing in at around a full pound. The body has filled out, adding muscle and bone along with more tissue. Your baby has translucent skin, through which all the myriad blood vessels are visible. Mothers may notice their baby kick and toss from side to side.

Your baby has also become covered with a substance called vernix caseosa. It resembles soft white cheese more than anything else. This covering protects your baby's skin while it's immersed in water for several months. Imagine what your skin would look like if you spent more than half the year in the bath.

Your uterus now reaches your belly button, and it's probably time to start thinking about maternity clothes. You might also start to experience heartburn and backaches. At the doctor's office, some more blood will be taken for a maternal serum screening—sometimes called multiple marker or triple screen for AFP (alpha-fetoprotein), HCG, and estriol. These tests can help indicate a possible risk of Down syndrome and neural-tube defects, such as spina bifida and anencephaly.

Your baby continues to instinctively swallow small amounts of amniotic fluid, and to recycle some of it as urine. Swallowing can give her hiccups, and you might even be able to feel her body jumping inside you. The baby tends to sleep during the day as you do your routine. When you lie down to relax, that's when she wakes up. Your baby already has high numbers of red blood cells, and infection-fighting white blood cells are beginning to be manufactured. Taste buds are starting to form on her tongue. The digestive system is now advanced enough to absorb water and sugar from the amniotic fluid.

Over the last few weeks, the motor neurons and the nerves connecting the muscles to the brain have grown into place, the spine has developed, and brain activity has increased noticeably. Your baby's movements are now consciously directed, and most of his or her senses are becoming active. The baby will become accustomed to the sound of blood rushing through the umbilical cord and to the sound of your heart beating, and will also become light sensitive.

You might get that strip running down your lower abdomen, and your nipples might look darker. Your blood volume has increased to meet the demands of pregnancy. The body is working overtime to nurture your baby, and may be leaving you fatigued. This mix of changes in your body, all spurred on by the release of different hormones, can make you feel a bit out of control. Things that didn't bother you before may leave you in tears.

Baby Needs Vitamin C and Iron

Vitamin C (also called citric acid) is going to become important right about now. You already know that vitamin C is good for fighting infections, but your body (and your baby's) also needs it to make collagen, which is the glue that holds your cells and tissues together.

Now that your baby is getting bigger, he or she is going to need more blood, too, and you need to supply it. More iron in your diet lets you build up your red blood cells.

You're also going to slowly start building a reserve—for lack of a better word—which will help when you suffer blood loss during the birth.

The Exercises

This trimester is where you're going to start noticing small changes in your body. The baby is starting to affect your posture, and your uterus has just enough mass to pinch veins and cause you some discomfort. So we'll be cutting way back on floor work and abdominal work. It won't be going away entirely, but don't expect to make any more advances. From here on in, it's just maintaining what you've got.

First off, use even less weight. At this point, for most of these exercises, you should not be using anything heavier than a five-pound weight, unless you've been training for quite a while with something much heavier.

The Routine

FIRST GROUP

Flys	3 to 5 pounds
Rear Shoulder	3 to 5 pounds
Side Bends	3 to 5 pounds
Squat on Bench	5 to 10 pounds

SECOND GROUP

Bench Pullover	5 to 10 pounds
Standing Row	5 to 10 pounds
Twist	5 pounds
Dead Lift	5 to 10 pounds

THIRD GROUP

Bicep Curls with a Twist	3 to 8 pounds
Kickback	3 to 5 pounds
Leg Lifts	
Stiff-Leg Dead Lift	5 to 10 pounds

For all these exercises, you're going to be doing five sets of five repetitions each. As before, work through each group before moving on to the next one.

Flys
pecs, biceps, lats

Lie down on your mat or bench with your arms stretched out to either side, so your body's shaped like the letter *T*. Your hands should be even with your shoulders. Inhale and lift the weights evenly, keeping your arms straight and pulling your chest down to help. Through this whole movement, your head and neck need to stay loose and relaxed—there's no reason for them to be tense during this exercise.

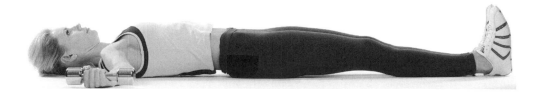

Finish with both arms straight, palms facing each other, and the weights touching above your chest. Exhaling, slowly let the weights back down, ending level with your shoulders. That's one repetition.

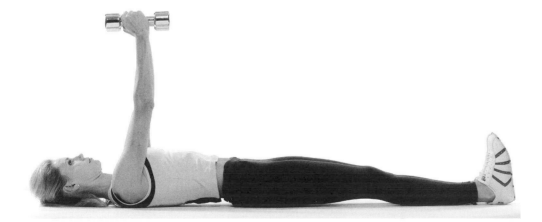

Rear Shoulder
triceps, deltoids, infraspinati, teres minor

Sit down on your bench or chair with your feet shoulders-width apart. Lean forward, keeping your back straight, so your belly settles between your thighs. Your arms should be at your sides, with the palms facing each other, so the weights are just hanging under your legs.

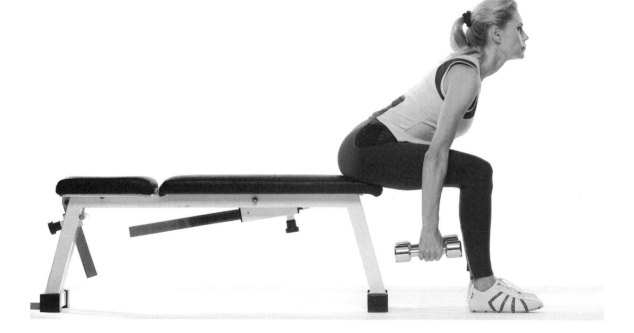

Inhaling, pull the weights up and out so they end at chest height. Don't go higher than your shoulders. Your arms stay bent, elbows high and palms back. Exhale and lower the dumbbells back beneath your thighs. That's one repetition.

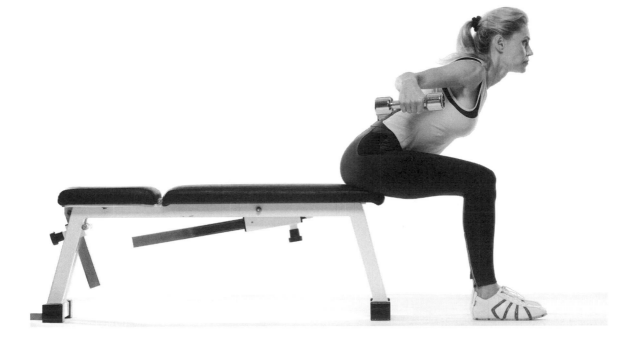

Side Bends
external obliques

Stand with your feet hips-width apart. Arms should be at your sides, holding the weights with palms facing in. Keep your chest out and chin up.

Bend your weight to the left, letting the left hand drop and the right hand rise. Stretch your left arm down until it reaches your knee, or the opposite weight is at your hip. Now relax and let your body come back to the center position.

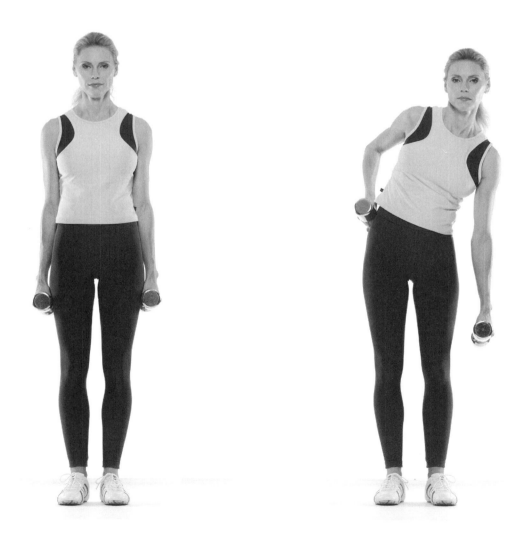

Once you're at center, pause and then bend to the right. Make sure to pause, so you're not just bobbing from side to side. Each time you come to center, that's one repetition.

The Side Bend exercise using small weights works the side muscles without putting too much strain on your body. When you are holding the weights and bending down, don't have too much weight, so as to avoid any strain on the stomach muscles. Listen to your body, connect with yourself, and feel every movement.

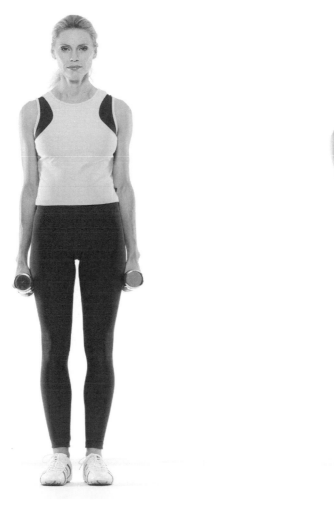
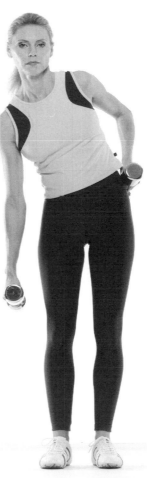

Squat on Bench
glutei maximi, semitendinosus solei, gastrocnemii, Achilles tendons

This exercise is very similar to the squat you've been doing already. We're just making a few adjustments.

Stand with your feet together and the bench behind you. Hold the weight in front of you with both hands, keeping your elbows as high as you can. This will help you not to lean forward when you squat.

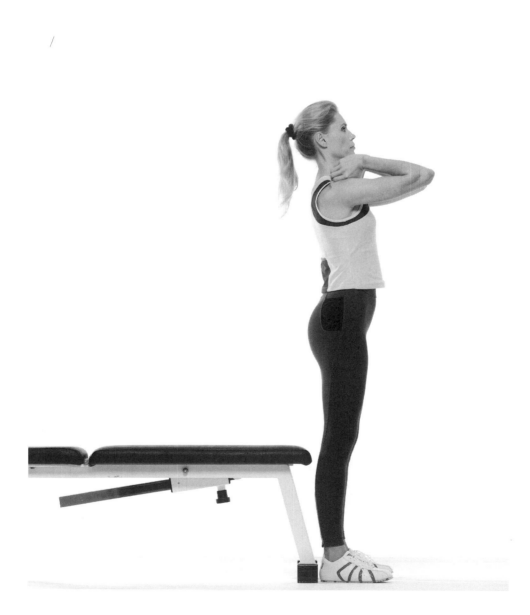

Inhale, tighten your abs, and squat. Keep your back straight, your chin and elbows up. Go all the way down until you're almost sitting on the bench.

Make your buttocks do the work, push back up from the heels (not your toes), and exhale. Remember, back straight chin up, elbows up. When you're standing straight, that's one repetition.

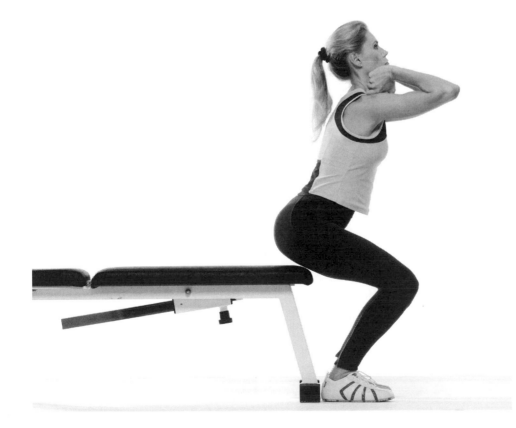

Bench Pullover
lats, pecs

This is a variation on the pullover we did in the last chapter.

Lie down on the bench, making sure to keep your abs tight and your lower back pushed against the bench. You don't want to arch your spine during this exercise.

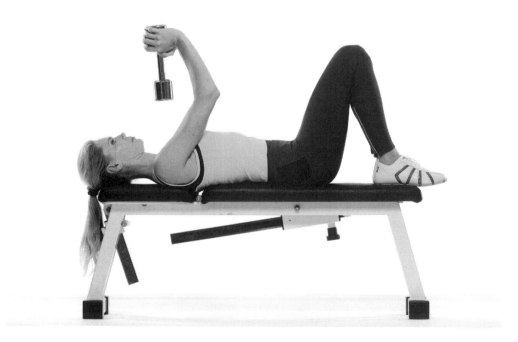

Hold one dumbbell in both hands about six inches over your solar plexus (the vee where your ribs come together above your stomach). Elbows should be bent and close to your body. Inhaling, lower the weight back until your arms straighten out "over" your head. Keep the dumbbell at that six-inch distance as you move, and don't let your elbows drift.

Bending your elbows and exhaling, bring the weight back over your head and down to the start position above your solar plexus. That's one repetition.

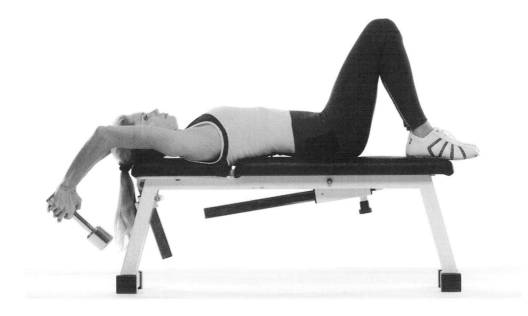

Standing Row

to give you strength in your upper back and rear shoulders, and to keep your flexibility in the upper chest and front deltoids

Start with feet together, chest out, and chin up. Arms should be straight out in front of you, just past your thighs, with your palms in.

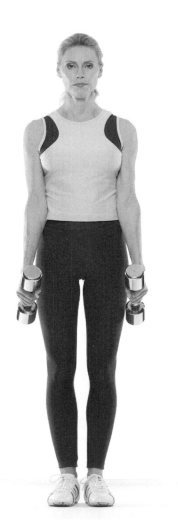

Inhaling, pull the weights up and back so they end up between your hips and your waist. Don't go higher than your waist. It's important to keep your arms moving in a straight line, so don't let your elbows drift—they should stay close to your body. Lower the weights, exhaling as you go. That's one repetition.

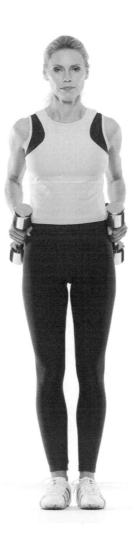

Twist
external obliques

Another easy one for you. Sit on a chair or at the end of a bench. Keep your abs tight, back straight, and rest the bar across your shoulders. If you don't have a bar, you can do this exercise with your hands placed behind your head.

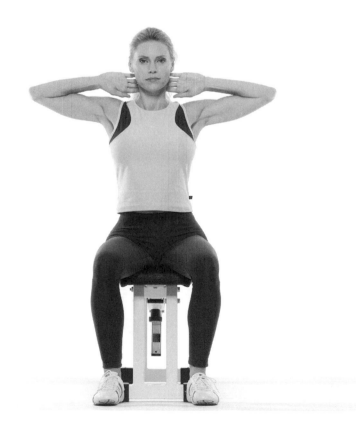

Keeping your chin up and chest out, rotate your body from side to side. Move from the waist, and make small movements (especially if you're using the bar). Each time you come back to center, that's one repetition.

Again, these are very small movements. If you feel any sort of pull on your stomach, you're turning too far.

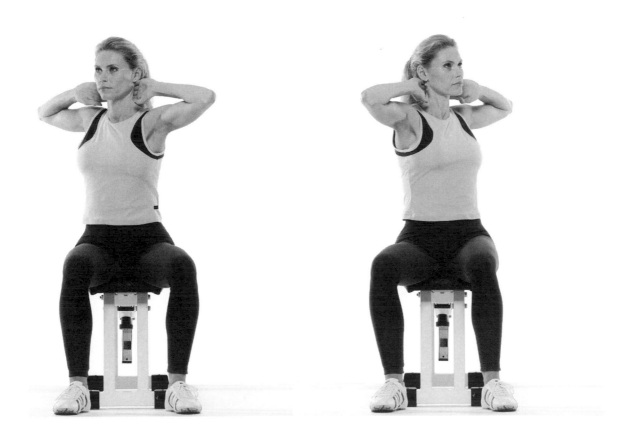

Dead Lift

gluteus maximus

This is the same exercise as in the previous chapter. The only difference is that we are going a little easier.

When you bend, only go down to your knees. There is no need to go lower.

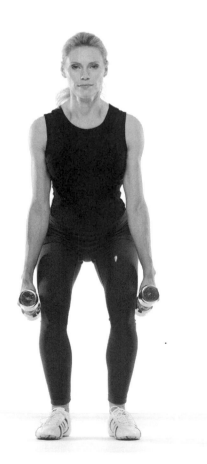

Hold your abs but keep your chest up while doing this movement. When coming back up, push yourself from your heels, come up on your toes, and exhale.

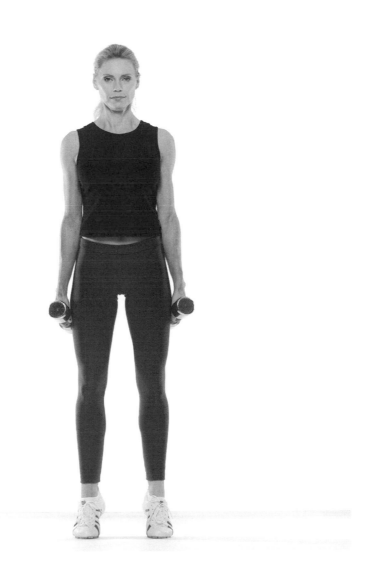

Bicep Curls with a Twist
biceps, brachioradiales

This works your entire biceps, which lets you keep everything balanced and proportional. Sit with your feet together. Keep your back straight, chest out, chin up. Arms straight at your sides, palms in.

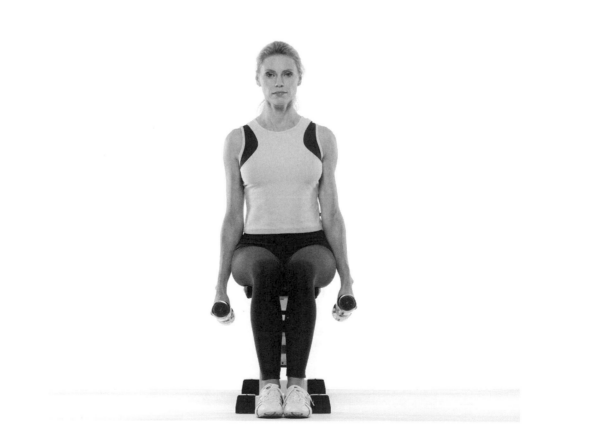

Inhale, tighten your abdominals, and lift the weights to your shoulders. As you do, turn your wrists so your palms are now facing your shoulders and the dumbbells are side to side. Now exhale and lower them to your sides, rotating your palms back as you do. You've just finished one repetition.

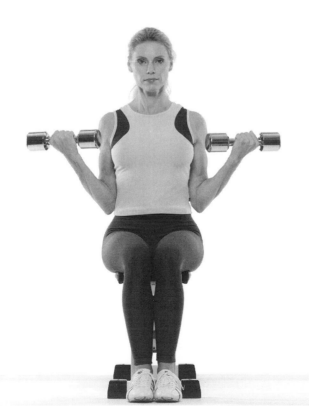

Kickback
triceps

Sit down on your bench or chair with your feet shoulders-width apart. Lean forward, keeping your chin up and back straight, so your belly settles between your legs. Your arms should be straight behind you, so your upper arm is parallel with the floor. Your forearm hangs down, holding the dumbbells with your palms in.

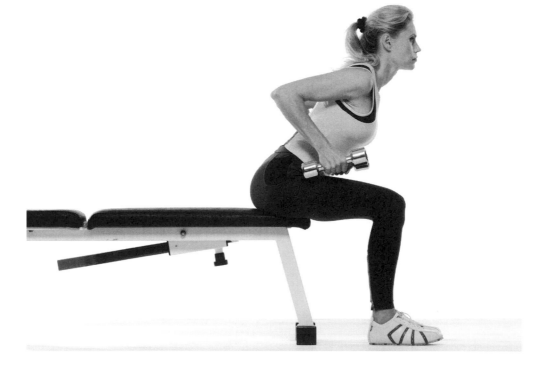

Inhale and lift your forearms until they lock with the weights straight behind you. Make sure your back stays flat. If you can't raise your arms all the way while keeping your spine straight, you need to use lighter weights.

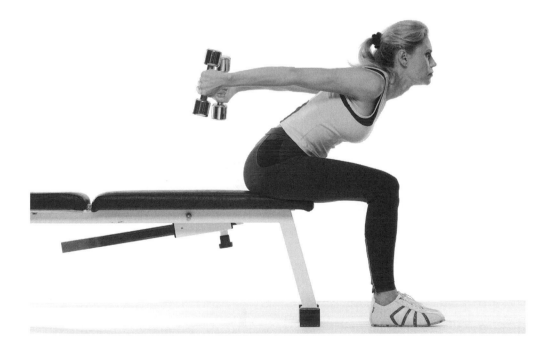

Leg Lifts
abdominals

Lie down on your bench (or on your floor mat). One of the most common mistakes in this exercise is letting your arms and neck tense up, so keep them relaxed. Put your hands under your buttocks to help angle them up and take pressure off your lower back.

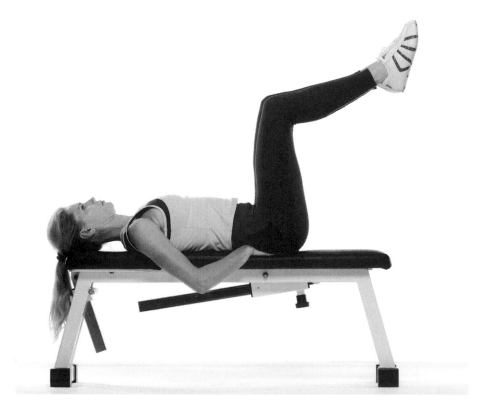

THE 30-MINUTE PREGNANCY WORKOUT BOOK

Lift your legs five inches off the bench. Keeping your back flat against the bench, inhale and slowly lift your legs using only your abdominals. Bend at the knees so you can raise your thighs easily to a vertical position.

Now, exhale and slowly lower your legs, stopping them five inches above the bench. This is one repetition.

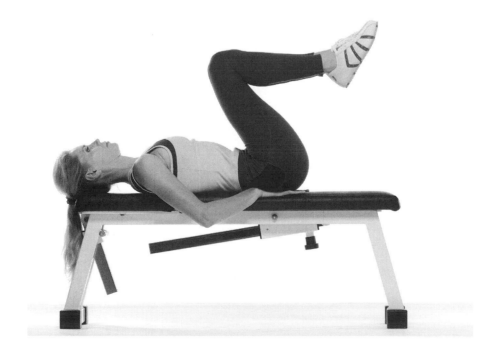

Stiff-Leg Dead Lift

glutei maximi, adductor magnus, semitendinosus solei, gastrocnemii, Achilles tendons; to increase the flexibility in the hamstring and lower back and buttocks

Stand with your feet hips-width apart, and bend from your hips down, keeping your back flat the whole time. Focus on keeping your back straight here; the object is not to go so low to the ground that your back bends.

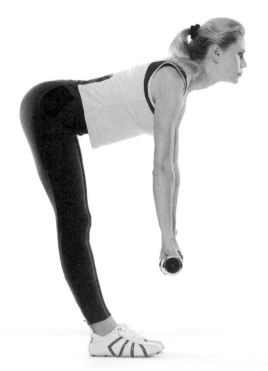

Rise up on your toes, make sure you're pushing from the heels and buttocks, and exhale. Repeat.

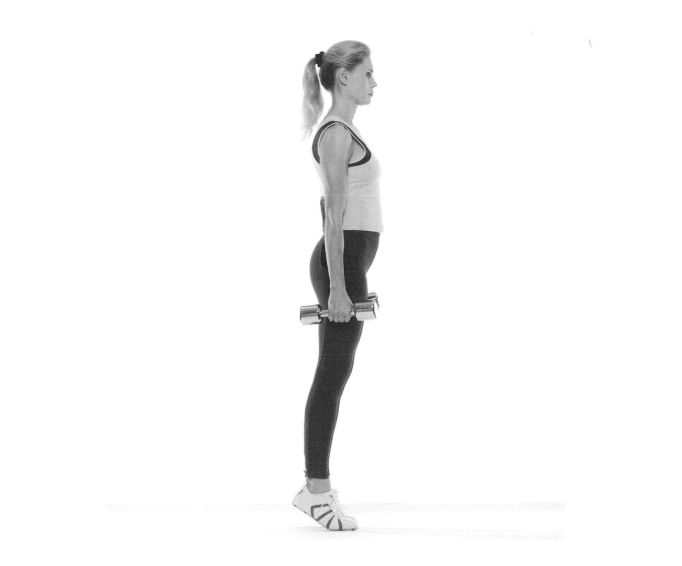

A Few More Notes

This trimester is all about transitions. Your fetus goes from being a tiny walnut to a recognizable baby over these three months. The changes in your body are becoming apparent, too.

It's going to be easy to overexert yourself now, because your boundaries and limitations are shifting and changing constantly. Watch your heart rate: It's getting higher at a rest state. That doesn't mean you can push it that much higher during your workouts. Keep an eye on your best friend, the heart monitor.

Go easy on yourself in all things.

4. The Third Trimester

The exercises featured in this chapter are:

Hammer

Triceps Extension

Shoulder Press

One-Arm Row

Reverse Hammer

Reverse Shoulder Press

Reverse One-Arm Row

Well, here is where it gets rough. Almost two-thirds of your weight gain is going to happen during this three-month period. Your baby barely weighs two pounds right now, but come the big day, she'll be close to seven.

The third trimester started well for me. Everything was running smooth, I had even fewer clients to deal with, and I found myself with more and more free time.

I'd been paging through some pregnancy magazines, always looking for more answers to more questions, when an advertisement caught my eye. A modeling agency in New York was looking for expectant mothers. Perfect, I thought. Pregnancy is such a beautiful thing, and I was perfectly qualified for the modeling part. I talked with the agency over the phone the next day, they gladly accepted me, and a week later they had me heading out to do a local commercial for the Gap.

When I arrived, however, my reception was less than enthusiastic. A heavyset woman pulled me aside to talk.

"There seems to have been a mistake," she told me.

"What's wrong?" I asked.

"You're...That is, we're looking for pregnant models," she said.

"I am pregnant," I replied.

"Well, yes," she said, nodding politely, "but we're looking for women who are much further along. You know, in their last trimester," she said.

"I'm almost in my eighth month," I said.

"Ahh." She frowned and waited another moment. "Well, I'm afraid you're just too skinny," she replied.

The moral of this story: If you want to do any pregnant modeling, throw this book away right now! It's such a common myth that you have to be heavy and unhealthy when you're pregnant that some people just won't accept anything else.

I did start to show a bit more over the next few weeks, and the modeling agency got me several print ads and a fashion show for Babystyle Clothing that was on KTLA News in Los Angeles. There was a cover photo shoot for *ePregnancy* magazine the day before Elli was born.

What You and Your Baby Are Doing

As you come into your last trimester, your baby is going to start growing quickly again. From here on in, she could be gaining as much as eight ounces every week. Her bone marrow has begun to produce her own blood cells, another sign the baby is getting ready to survive outside the womb. The brain continues to develop, and the baby's senses have become fully active. She's actually looking around, feeling your heartbeat, and hearing your voice now.

By this point in the pregnancy, some women will be having difficulty moving around. Even eating may be difficult because the baby is crowding your stomach and intestines. You will still be able to exercise until the day of labor, but you'll probably slow down the pace of your workouts. Listen to your body and rest a lot.

You may also begin to experience Braxton-Hicks contractions (a tightening of the uterus) which can last up to two minutes. These aren't exactly painful, but they can be annoyingly intense. Fat deposits continue to build throughout, and now your baby is large enough for her presentation to be determined. This is the orientation in the womb, which either is breech (bottom) or head first.

Pregnancy is about more than just physical changes. No matter how happy you are about your baby, feelings of stress and anxiety are as common as excitement and anticipation. Moms may experience mood swings. You don't always feel attractive, but go easy on yourself. Remember to talk to your spouse and to your friends. They'll remind you that you're beautiful and wonderful—if they know what's good for them....

As you enter your eighth month, you may be able to detect the shape of a head, foot, or elbow through your abdomen. Finger- and toenails have developed, and so has the beginning of an immune system (some of which she's gotten right from you) in her blood. Your baby should have settled into her birth position. By the end of this month, he or she is about eighteen inches long and weighs as much as six pounds.

If the baby were born now, her lungs would probably work, but she would still need to be in an incubator to stay warm enough. If an early delivery is likely, doctors will test lung maturity with an amniocentesis procedure that checks levels of surfactant.

Over the last few weeks, your baby has been building up waste material in his or her intestines. It's a greenish-black substance called meconium, and it's made up of broken-down red blood cells, cells shed by her intestinal lining, mucus, bile, and even skin cells and lanugo she's shed into the amniotic fluid and then swallowed. Meconium will be the first waste your baby passes after birth.

Drink a lot of water to prevent constipation, and eat small meals to avoid heartburn. You may need to urinate frequently. The top of the uterus has probably reached its highest point, making breathing a bit uncomfortable.

There may be a lot of motion now. Your little one has lungs he or she is trying to work with, limbs to move, hands to grab with, and they're all new and exciting. This is normal, so don't be unnerved by the activity. The baby will slip down into position for birth sometime during the last month, and that will make your heartburn and shortness of breath let up. You will feel more pressure on your groin and bladder, though.

At this time, you are probably exhausted due to your many discomforts. Your breasts may even be leaking colostrum (a yellow, watery precursor of breast milk). If your baby is in a breech position, your physician may want to discuss the possibility of turning the baby or of performing a C-section. There's also a check for group B streptococcus (GBS), a common genital bacterium that can be passed to the baby during delivery and cause severe illness (or even death) if it's present. Prior to delivery, your doctor will take a culture for testing, and if it's positive, intravenous antibiotics are administered during labor.

Toxemia is an old term, sometimes used interchangeably with preeclampsia, one of the hypertensive disorders of pregnancy. It literally means "poison in the blood" and it's another potentially serious complication in later pregnancy. Symptoms include high blood pressure, rapid weight gain due to edema (swelling), and protein in the urine. Untreated, toxemia can lead to seizures and coma and death of an infant.

Your baby may seem much less active as the birth approaches, but you shouldn't worry. This stillness is because she's finally gotten too big for the womb. The umbilical cord is half an inch thick and may be knotted or wrapped around the baby. A few of your antibodies will also cross the placenta barrier and enter your baby's bloodstream, giving his or her immune system a temporary boost to help until it gets into full swing. The average baby will be twenty inches long and about seven and a half pounds by this point.

Final preparations are being made for birth, which could safely take place at any time now. Pack your hospital bag, and keep an eye out for signs of imminent labor. Watch for fluid leaking from your vagina; this is your amniotic sac or water breaking. Blood discharge could be the mucus plug in your cervix giving way.

Healthy Eating and Nutrition

Your baby's brain develops the most in the last trimester, so it's important you've got a good supply of protein coming in. Those essential amino acids we mentioned earlier in the book will be used for nerve cells and brain tissue.

You've known that calcium helps build strong teeth and bones. Well, now your baby needs to build up her bones, too. Remember, if you're not taking in enough calcium, the baby will pull from your storage and weaken your own bones, especially if you're older.

You're going to need even more iron this trimester. The baby is starting to make her own blood supply now, and so she needs to start building her own stores of iron. Again, if you're not giving it to her, she'll take it where she can find it.

The Exercises

I'd often see pregnant women in the club, with their pregnant trainers who were charging one hundred dollars a day, and they were both so out of shape. It stunned me. How can a trainer be instructing someone, inspiring someone, when she can't even take care of herself? They'd all ask me, "You look so good, what are you doing differently?"

The big difference, of course, was that I was actually training, not just going to the club so I could say I'd been training. Many of the other expectant women at the gym— the clients and the trainers—were uninspired and unhappy, and they'd drag each other down with their negativity. I'd try to help, but I found that quite often it wasn't welcome. They'd made a choice for the path they wanted to follow, and now they weren't willing to accept a change.

If you feel yourself slipping into one of those cycles, stop and think about all that negative energy going to your baby. At this point in your pregnancy, he or she can actually hear and feel you, knows your tones, your moods, and can sense tension levels. What kind of input are you giving your baby?

Your workout should be simple. Don't think you have to put a ton of effort into it to accomplish something. These exercises are small and simple, so have fun with them.

At this point, you're probably having trouble bending over, so most of the workout is going to concentrate on the upper body. This new group of exercises is sometimes called a Super Set, because it helps blast out your arm muscles.

Super Set

FIRST GROUP		SECOND GROUP	
Hammer	3 pounds	Shoulder Press	3 pounds
Triceps Extension	6 pounds	One-Arm Row	6 pounds

THIRD GROUP		FOURTH GROUP	
Reverse Hammer	3 pounds	Reverse Shoulder Press	3 pounds
Triceps Extension	6 pounds	Reverse One-Arm Row	6 pounds

All we're doing now is three sets of ten each. These should be quick and easy, and they're another example of lifting weights as a cardio exercise. The weights are really low now, and they should feel comfortable enough that you can do the routine and keep up a good pace.

In the third trimester of pregnancy, the focus should be on the upper body. You don't want to put any extra weight on the lower part of the body, especially the legs. By working with low weights this becomes more of a cardio exercise that will increase your upper body strength, make you lean, and also help prepare your back for the time when you'll be carrying your newborn.

New mothers often complain about their extra upper body weight while nursing their babies. The breasts will have doubled in size because of the milk they now carry. And the extra weight gained from the pregnancy will put a strain on their back if they skip the recommended upper body workouts.

The upper body workouts will not only prevent you from feeling back strain, but will stop you from hunching forward when nursing your baby as well.

After doing the Super Set, I also like to spend about thirty minutes on a stationary bike. It's low impact and helps to keep blood flowing in the legs. This is important, because you're very susceptible to blood clots at the last stage of pregnancy. Clots are painful and hard to get rid of once you get them, so you want to keep your legs active during these few months. I ended up with two blood clots in my right leg during pregnancy, and it was not pretty. I had to wear support hose and spent a lot of my free time with my leg elevated.

Make sure you use an upright bike, not a recumbent one that lets you lean back and pedal with your feet in a higher position. (This will put more pressure on your back and pinch off the vena cava.)

Hammer
to increase the strength in the triceps and biceps

Stand with your feet hips-width apart, keep your chest up.

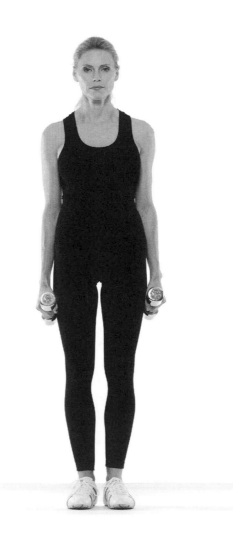

Fire your arms straight up over your head in one movement, let the weights drop back to the starting position, and allow your arms to stay close to your body so that the movement is as straight as possible. Exhale.

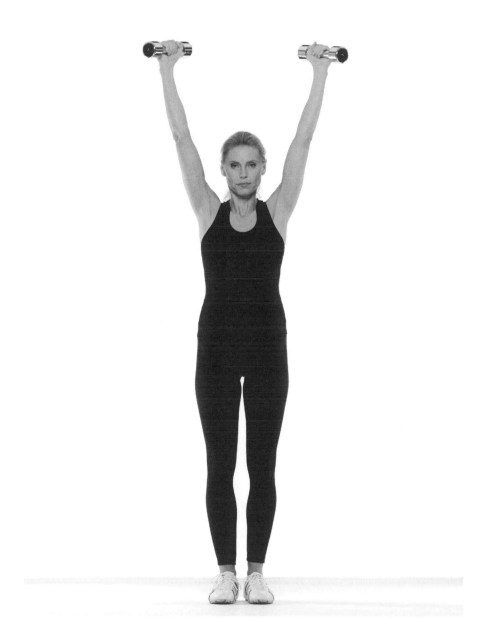

Triceps Extension
to strengthen the triceps and give flexibility to thoracic spine and rib cage

Stand with feet hips-width apart, and hold the weights in both hands behind you, hanging vertically. Allow your elbows to stay close to the side of your head and inhale.

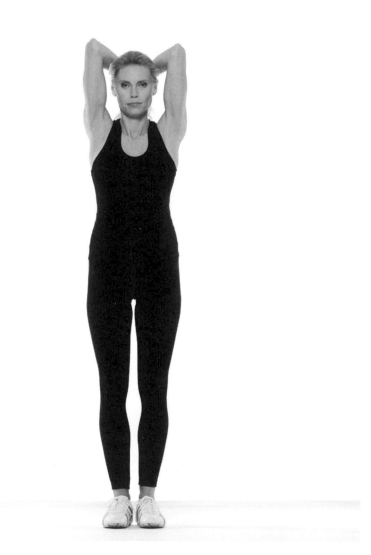

Lift the weight up above your head in a straight line. Make sure your elbows stay close to your ears when you come down, and exhale.

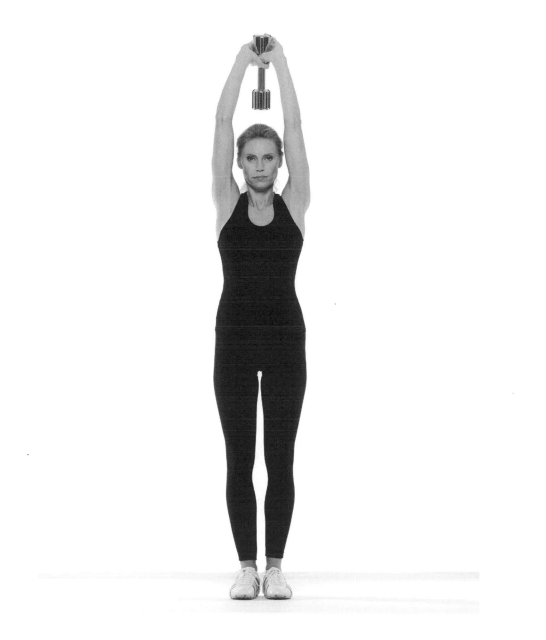

Shoulder Press
deltoids, lats, pecs

This exercise is, essentially, half a hammer. Start with your feet hips-width apart, your chest out, and your chin up. Your arms should be bent up at the elbow, so the weights are sitting in front of your shoulders, palms in.

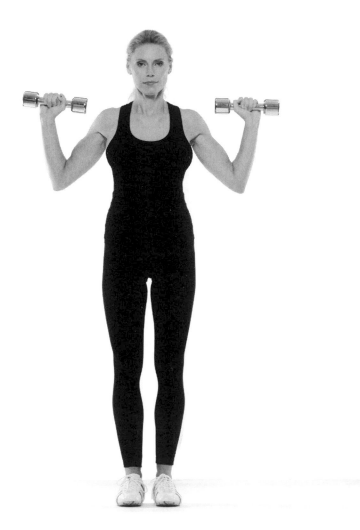

Now, inhale, keep your abs tight, and exhale as you push the weights up to the ceiling, straightening your arms. While pushing up, pull down with your chest.

Let the weights drop back down to the start position, exhaling as you do. You've just completed one repetition.

Remember to keep your spine straight through all of this. Also, keep the weights with your palms always facing out through the whole exercise.

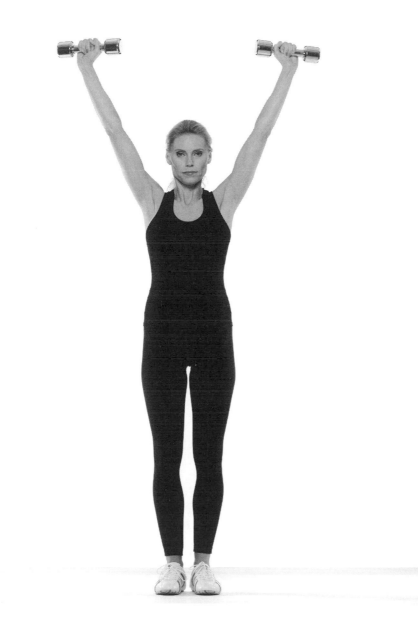

One-Arm Row
lats, triceps

Stand with your feet a bit more than hips-width apart. You may have to go even wider, depending on where your belly is right now. Bend from the hips, using your left hand on a chair or bench for balance, until your back is parallel with the floor. Make sure your back is straight and flat, and your head and spine line up. As always, don't go down past the point that you can't keep your back straight.

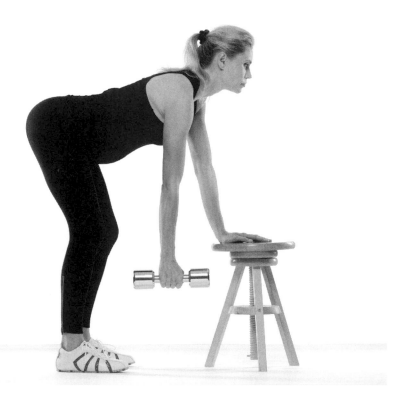

Let your right arm hang free with the weight held palm-in. Inhale and pull your elbow back, lifting the dumbbell straight back to the inside of your hip. Keep your arms tight to your body and your palms turned in. Exhale as you let the weight back down, and, once your arm is straight, switch hands. That's one repetition.

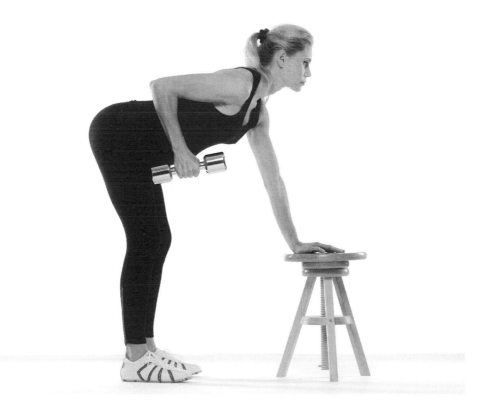

Reverse Hammer

to increase strength in your deltoids, triceps, and pecs

Stand with feet hips-width apart. Inhale, keeping your stomach tight.

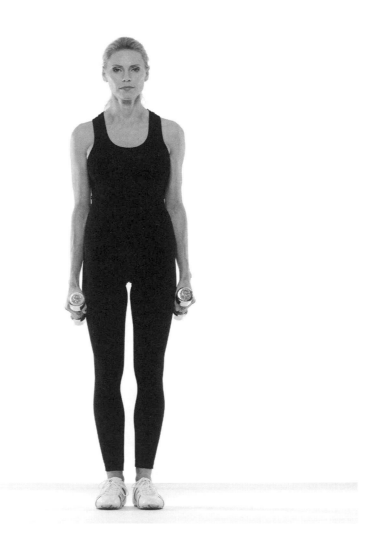

Fire the weights straight up and twist your palms at your shoulder. Continue firing straight up, let your weights drop back to the starting position, and make sure your arms stay close to your body. Exhale.

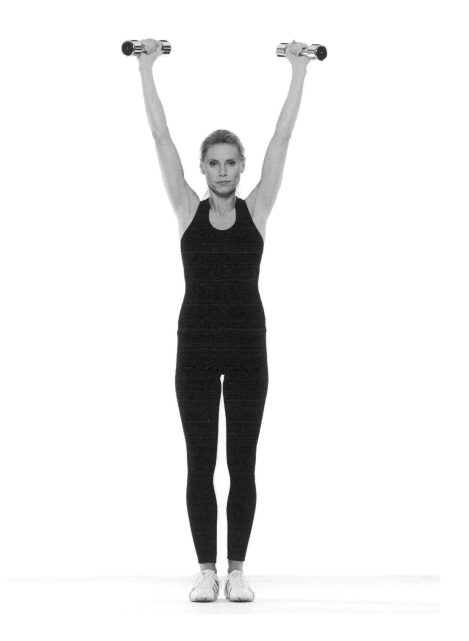

Triceps Extension
to strengthen the triceps and give flexibility to thoracic spine and rib cage

Stand with feet hips-width apart, hold the weights in both hands behind you, hanging vertically. Allow your elbows to stay close to the side of your head and inhale.

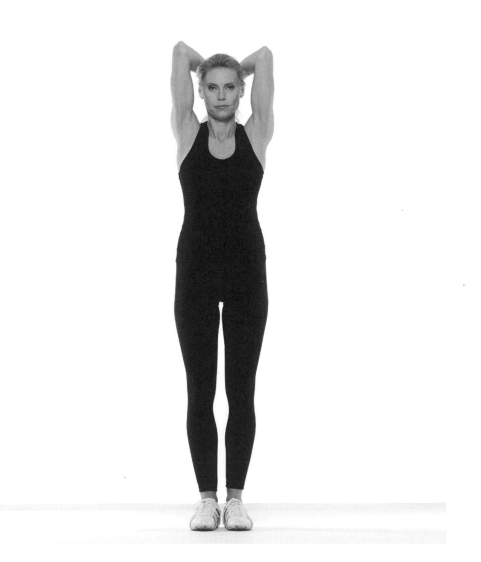

Lift the weight up above your head in a straight line. Make sure your elbows stay close to your ears when you come down. Exhale.

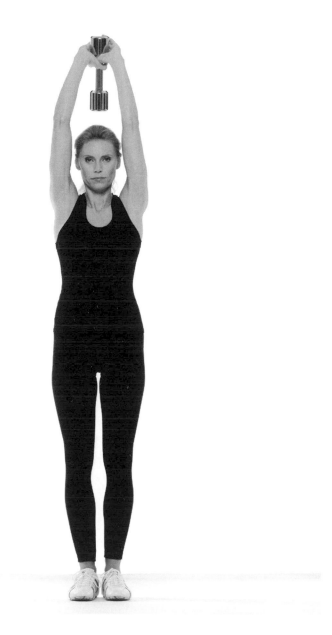

Reverse Shoulder Press
biceps, deltoids, pecs, lats

Like most of the "reverse" exercises, this one involves just a slight change. Start with your feet hips-width apart, your chest out, and your chin up. Your arms should be bent up at the elbow, so the dumbbells are sitting slightly wider than, and out from, your shoulders, palms out.

Now, inhale, keep your abs tight, and exhale as you fire the weights to the ceiling, straightening your arms. While pushing up, pull down your chest.

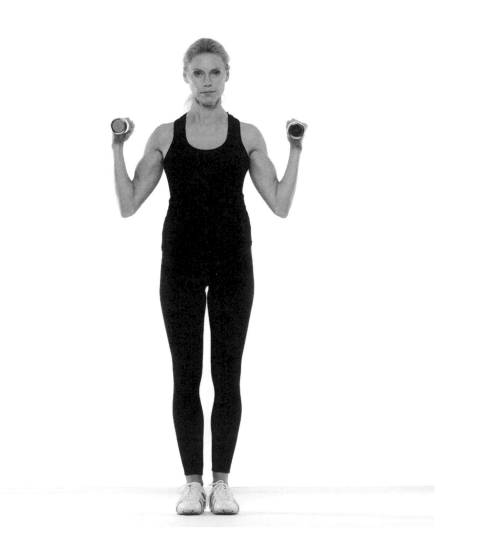

Let the weights drop back down to the start position, exhaling as you do. You've just completed one repetition.

Remember to keep your spine straight through all of this. Also, keep the weights with your palms always facing each other through the whole exercise (just like with the Hammer).

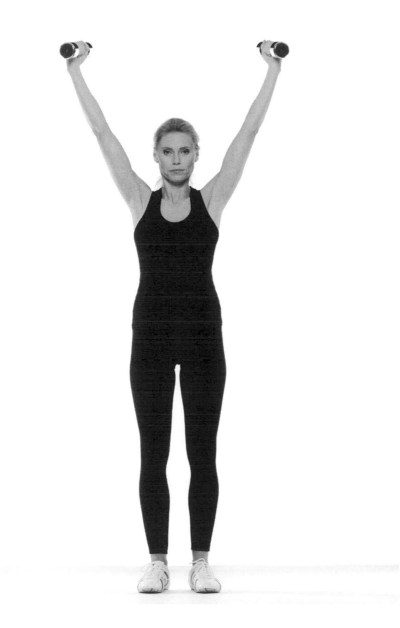

Reverse One-Arm Row
lats, triceps

Like the Reverse Shoulder Press, this exercise is almost the same as the One-Arm Row, with a minor tweak to isolate a different set of muscles.

Stand with your feet a bit more than hips-width apart. Bend from your hips, resting your left hand on the chair or bench, until your back is parallel with the floor. Make sure your back is straight and flat, and your head and spine are lined up.

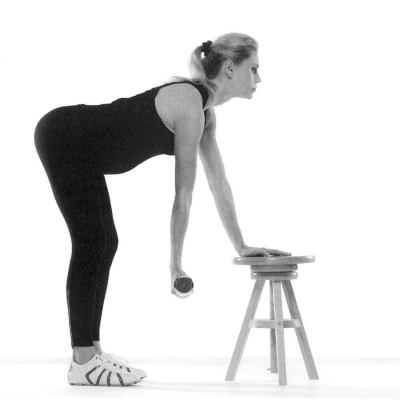

Let your right arm hang free with the weight held from side to side, palm out. Inhale and pull your elbow back, lifting the dumbbell straight back to the inside of your hip. Keep your arms tight to your body, and the weight side to side. Exhale as you let the weight back down, and once your arm is straight, switch hands. That's one repetition.

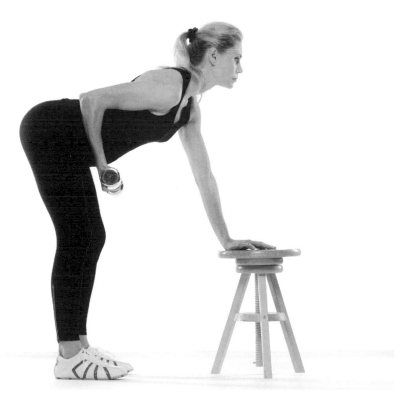

A big destroyer of the body and its muscles is the constant repetition or movement that a person performs over the course of a day. People sitting at a desk doing the same repetitive hand movement with a computer mouse are doing damage to themselves unless they break the cycle with regular exercise routines. It is very easy for a pregnant woman to make excuses and neglect her exercises because she is in an altered state. It's been proven that if a pregnant woman is more alert and in good shape, she will have a smoother delivery and a faster recovery time postlabor. And a happy, fit pregnant woman will mean an equally happy, healthy baby. An unborn baby feels everything, and a pregnant woman should not become upset or be engaged in arguments. That will only distress the baby.

A Few More Notes

So, this is it. Everything in this chapter will be with you until that last day. Or the first day, depending on how you look at it.

There's one thing to mention here: airplanes. Most pregnant women can travel without experiencing unusual symptoms or it having an adverse effect on their pregnancies, according to the American College of Obstetricians and Gynecologists. There are some instances in which air travel is not recommended, though. Women who have medical or obstetrical complications, such as pregnancy-induced hypertension, poorly controlled diabetes, sickle-cell disease, or other conditions that could result in an emergency medical situation probably should not fly while they're pregnant. Most airlines prefer women not to travel after their thirty-sixth week because of the risks of going into labor.

5. The Birth

I t was a Friday in mid-October when I returned from my morning workout at the gym and got a call from Dr. Katz's office. I'd had to cancel an appointment the day before because of a photo shoot, and they were trying to reschedule. He wanted to make sure I got in my weekly exam, especially now that we were getting so close to my due date.

"Today might not be good," his assistant told me. "He's in surgery all day," she said.

"That's no problem. I can come in on Monday," I answered.

"Okay. Just let me confirm that with him," she said. She put me on hold for a moment and then said, "Anna, he'd prefer to see you first thing today, before he goes into surgery."

When I was at the office, Dr. Katz ran an ultrasound test and discovered the amniotic fluid levels in my womb were almost nonexistent.

"We're going to have to do a cesarean section to deliver the baby," said Dr. Katz. "It's just too risky."

I was caught off guard, but I had been prepared for the possibility of a cesarean since we discovered she was a breech baby. We'd even gone ahead and scheduled the operation a few days earlier, but hearing Dr. Katz say it out loud just seemed a bit final.

"Are you sure nothing could change between now and then?" I asked him. He shook his head. "Not *then*, Anna," he told me. "We're going to perform the C-section today. Like I said, it's too risky to let it go for another two weeks."

I'm not going to bore you with what happened over the next few hours. I had to wait for my breakfast to digest before they could wheel me into the delivery room. But in the end, it was all worth it. That was the day I finally got to meet my daughter, Elli, face-to-face.

Cesarean Delivery

The reasons for a cesarean vary. You might not be able to deliver vaginally because your pelvis is an unusual shape or disproportionate to the size of the baby's head, or if you have placenta previa, an active herpes infection, or your baby is in a difficult breech position. Sometimes you may require it because your labor is not progressing well, or if your baby is in distress.

You'll be given either an epidural or spinal anesthetic. Both will numb the lower part of your body (from hips down). Sometimes a general anesthetic is administered with an intravenous drip while a catheter is inserted into your bladder to empty it. Antibiotics are given to those experiencing preterm labor or who have a fever during labor.

A small dividing screen will be placed across your upper body so you cannot see the operation. Your partner can sit near your head so he can give you emotional support and hold your hand. Your abdomen will be covered with antiseptic to kill off any bacteria on the skin, and your pubic hair will be shaved. A low transverse skin incision will be made through your abdomen wall, and then through your uterus. You may feel a sensation of uncomfortable pressure. After an initial examination, your baby will be handed to you. The placenta will be removed and examined, and your incision will be stitched up.

After the birth, you'll be taken into the recovery room for a couple of hours. Meanwhile, the baby is taken to the nursery for different medical checks. Then the baby will be returned to you, and you can start breast-feeding and begin bonding with your child. It will take a few weeks to fully recover from the operation.

If you have a cesarean, you'll be required to stay in the hospital for a few days after the surgery. It may be difficult to sit or stand straight, and it'll hurt when you cough or laugh.

There's not much else I can tell you here that your doctor hasn't already discussed, but I would like to address one other point.

After delivery, your doctor will clamp and cut the umbilical cord. The cord is either discarded with the placenta as biological waste, or the doctor can use a syringe to remove the blood that remains in the cord. The process does not affect your baby, and it won't have any effect on the birthing procedure.

Cord blood contains stem cells, which are useful for numerous medical treatments, including cancers, blood disorders, and heart disease. Banking this blood saves the cells in case your baby ever needs them in the future. In general, you will pay an enrollment fee, processing fee, and then an annual storage fee afterwards, but the fees vary from registry to registry.

If you can't afford to bank your child's cord blood, or don't feel compelled to keep the blood for your family, you may choose to donate it to a public bank. It doesn't cost anything to preserve the cord blood, and it may help somebody else who needs it.

Ten Motivational Tips

1. You are what you eat, so eat smart. You are what you think, so think smart.

2. It's not how many hours you put in, but how much you put in those hours.

3. Happiness is not doing what you like, but liking what you do.

4. Hard times don't last; strong people do.

5. We make a living by what we get. We make a life by what we give.

6. The secret of success is to start from scratch and keep on scratching.

7. We see obstacles when we take our eyes off our goals.

8. Begin where you are, but don't stay where you are.

9. Winners believe they can.

10. If it were not for hopes, the heart would break.

A Few More Notes

One of the many doctors I am impressed with is Dr. Stuart McGill, a professor of spine biomechanics at the University of Waterloo in Waterloo, Ontario, Canada, who is also the chair of the Department of Kinesiology. He has advised governments, corporations, and even elite athletes on health and fitness issues, and on how to correct some serious back ailments. He is the author of *Ultimate Back Fitness and Performance* (Wabuno Publishers), and to get more information on him you can visit his Web site: www.backfitpro.com.

In his book, Dr. McGill says that he has seen too many people develop bad backs in an effort to increase their fitness level. That should not be the case. He said that building strength and function is sometimes very difficult for those who follow the traditional approach, practiced in the United States and dominated by bodybuilding concepts. He said that building muscle strength is an easy component to enhance the foundation fundamentals of healthy motion and motion patterns, joint stability, and endurance. When you achieve that solid foundation, then serious strength with speed and power will follow.

Dr. McGill has devised a five-stage program that builds the ultimate back with core strength on a foundation that has strength, speed, and power training.

The five-stage program includes

1. Groove motion patterns, motor patterns with corrective exercise

2. Building whole body and joint stability (with super stiffness)

3. Increasing endurance

4. Building strength

5. Developing power, agility

What else can I say? This is the day you've been waiting for, and working toward, for the past nine months. Congratulations!

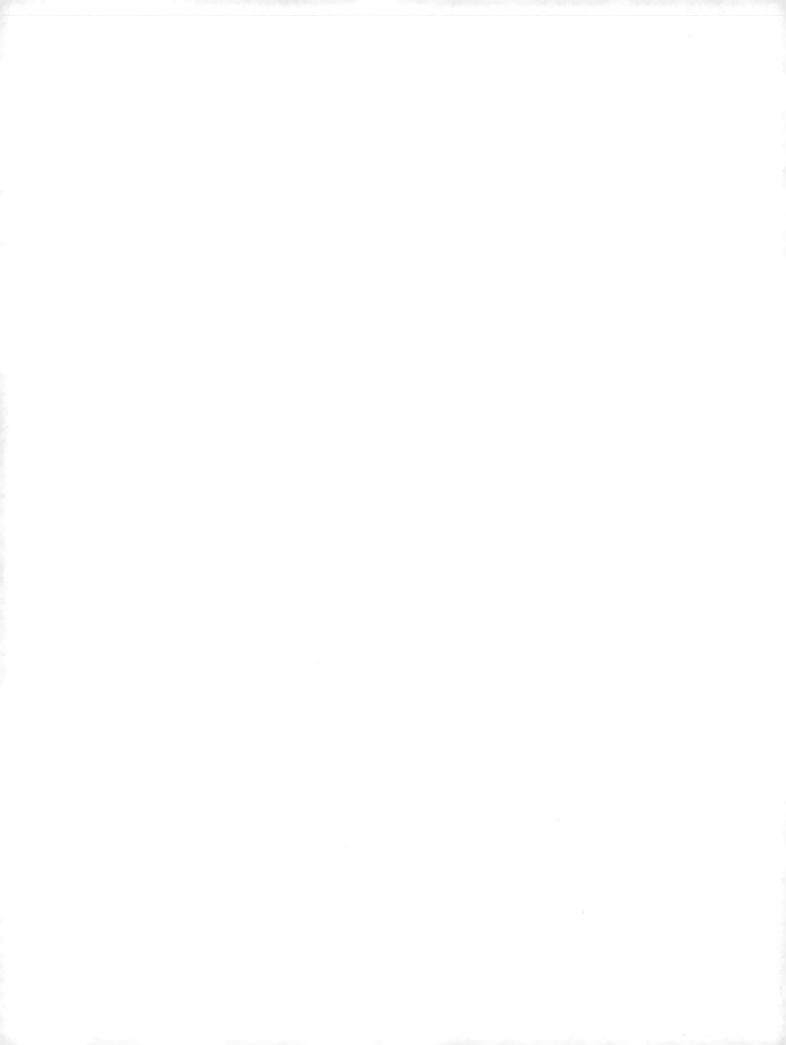

6. The Recovery

One of the downsides to being in shape before the birth was that I was up and ready to go less than a week after Elli was born. I wanted to go back to the gym, but Dr. Katz had other ideas. It was more than six weeks before my abdomen healed from the surgery enough that I could go back to a daily workout.

Interestingly, my body fat in December 2001 (before I was pregnant) was 17.9 percent; then in April 2002, after doing my Olympic weight lifting program, my body fat dropped to 11.7 percent. This was remarkable, because at the time I was three months pregnant! I am convinced my body fat decreased due to the fact I was performing the Olympic weight lifting training program.

The weights that I had used burned the fat, "leaned" me out, and gave definition to my entire body. I was doing the program three times a week, as recommended, and I incorporated it with the Routine and the Super Set program. Normally, if I had not done the Olympic training beforehand, there is no doubt that my body fat would have gone up when I became pregnant, because I would have been eating a lot more. My baby, Elli, was born October 18, 2002, and three months later, my body fat was only 15.1 percent, back to the point I was almost at previously.

What You and Your Baby Are Doing

Well, guess what? You're a mom now.

The more in touch you are with you baby, the more your feelings will grow, and the happier and healthier your baby will be. It's very important to be involved in your baby's care right from the start, while you are in the hospital. Breast-feeding is an ideal way to give love to your newborn baby. If you are having problems, ask for a lactation consultant.

After the past nine months, all leading up to the actual trauma of giving birth to your baby, it's not unusual to feel drained, perhaps even lessened. Postpartum depression is a form of depression that occurs in some women after childbirth. Those physical and emotional stresses are usually accompanied by a lack of rest and a wave of hormonal changes that can affect emotions even further. At this point, caring for a new baby may seem overwhelming.

General symptoms of depression can include appetite problems, decreased energy, feeling very sensitive emotionally, irritability, loss of motivation, withdrawal, low self-esteem, pessimism, and negativity. Untreated postpartum depression interferes with bonding between mother and infant.

The two most common ways of treating serious depression are with antidepressant medication and with psychotherapy.

Healthy Eating and Nutrition

A combination of healthy eating and regular exercise is the best way to lose any leftover pregnancy weight. No crash diets are allowed. If you are breast-feeding, it's important to eat healthy and to get the extra calories you need for adequate milk production. Ask your practitioner what the best daily caloric intake is for you.

Vitamin A is going to be important again. I mentioned earlier that it helps repair and rebuild tissue. Well, now you're the one who needs work. This vitamin A is all for you as you rebuild tissues along the vagina and uterus that were damaged during the birth.

Don't forget to drink plenty of fluids, particularly if you're breast-feeding and especially if you're exercising, too.

The Exercises

You should wait to exercise until after your postpartum checkup (about six weeks after the birth). Your doctor can examine you and let you know when it's safe to resume your exercise program. Having workout equipment at home helps, too, even if it's just a few dumbbells. Try to squeeze in some time for working out while your baby is sleeping.

Exercise is good for mental health as well as for your physical conditioning. Try not to get discouraged with the additional demands that new motherhood brings.

Okay, the exercises you do are going to vary depending on how the birth went. If you had a regular birth, you're going to do the Time Trial from chapter 2. I'll list it here for you again:

Time Trial

Hammer	3 to 5 pounds
Triceps Extension	8 to 10 pounds
Crunches	
Dead Lift	8 to 10 pounds

SECOND GROUP

Standing Fly	3 to 5 pounds
Standing Row	5 to 8 pounds
Stiff-Leg Dead Lift	5 to 8 pounds
Crunches (straight leg)	

THIRD GROUP

Reverse Hammer	3 to 5 pounds
Side Crunches	
Pullover	5 to 8 pounds
Front Squat	8 to 10 pounds

Unlike during the first trimester, though, you're going to do only two sets of eight reps for these exercises. Watch your weights, also. Your body has just been through a very traumatic experience involving lots of blood loss. You need to be aware and to be cautious. Turn to chapter 2 for detailed instructions.

If you had a cesarean, you're probably in even worse shape, but for different reasons. You're not going to be able to do anything with your abdominals for at least two months. So, for now, all that's safe for you to do is the Super Set from chapter 4. I'll list that again, too.

Super Set

FIRST GROUP		SECOND GROUP	
Hammer	3 pounds	Shoulder Press	3 pounds
Triceps Extension	6 pounds	One-Arm Row	6 pounds
THIRD GROUP		FOURTH GROUP	
Reverse Hammer	3 pounds	Reverse Shoulder Press	3 pounds
Triceps Extension	6 pounds	Reverse One-Arm Row	6 pounds

As with the Time Trial, you're going to do only two sets of eight reps each. Keep in mind that you're doing only the Super Set from chapter 4. Don't try to get on the exercise bike. Turn to chapter 4 for detailed instructions.

Now that you've got those down, let's talk about Kegel exercises. You may have heard of them already, in relation to childbirth, sex, or even bladder problems. They're named after Dr. Arnold Kegel, who developed them, and they're very, very easy to do.

Lie down on your mat on your back. Your feet should be pulled in and your knees up. Press your hands down on your pubic muscles, just above your vagina. These are the muscles you use to "hold it" when you need to go to the bathroom.

Squeeze your muscles hard, and then slowly tighten your abdominals, rolling your body forward and up as if you were doing a crunch. Try to hold this pose for ten seconds. Now relax your muscles, settling back down to the mat. That's one repetition.

You want to do these until your pubic muscles are exhausted. How many times that is depends on what kind of shape you're in, but everyone should be able to manage at least ten.

Remember, if you had a cesarean section, you won't be able to do Kegels for at least two months after the birth, possibly longer. Don't rush into them and hurt yourself. Just wait; then add them on to the end of your workout.

A Few More Notes

Well, you did it. You made it through nine months and managed to look good the whole time, keeping healthy and strong for you and your baby. Hopefully you'll want to take what you've learned here and apply it to the rest of your life.

This is a time of recovery, so don't be scared to relax a little bit. Your body needs to rest and recover, and that is a natural, healthy step for it. In a few weeks, your doctor will give you the okay to start exercising again.

Some Last Thoughts

While I was pregnant, I soaked up all sorts of information. There was just so much new material for me, far more than I could ever fit in a book the size you're reading now. Some things I do want to mention don't quite fit in anywhere else in this book.

Studies have isolated three distinct phases that women go through during pregnancy. These phases are referred to as developmental tasks. First, you have to accept the fact of your pregnancy. Second, you come to feel the baby as a part of your own body. Third, you release the baby from your body through childbirth.

Learning You Are Pregnant

When a woman announces to her partner that she is pregnant, it is a life-changing moment. It's up to the partner to be helpful as much as possible to the pregnant spouse by doing the following: Encourage her by telling her she is still beautiful. Accept the fact and see her pregnancy as a thing of beauty and not anything else. Be willing to do things for the pregnant spouse, such as prepare the nursery, do some of the household chores, and do things together, including accompany her to the doctor's office.

The partner should try to understand a pregnant woman's mood swings and be patient, helpful, and cooperative. Often the partner can feel excluded and not involved in the raising of the baby, so the mother must try and bring her partner in as much as she can.

Pregnancy also starts a new phase of your relationship with your partner. Impending parenthood may bring shock and euphoria that can last awhile. Your spouse may also need some emotional and physical distance from you, and from the reality of the pregnancy, in order to sort out feelings. These are all normal behaviors.

Ironically, sex is often the first thing out the window after a couple creates the ultimate expression of their love and has a baby. Your interest in sex may change throughout your pregnancy, due to nausea, hormones, and plain old fatigue. Even if an expectant mother isn't interested in sex, a couple can still share intimacy. Communication is vital, and you are mature enough to share a child, so be honest with each other about your feelings.

Vaginal intercourse can be continued as usual if your pregnancy is uncomplicated. Sex will not cause any problems. The fetus floats safely in a cushion of amniotic fluid and will not be harmed by a bumping of the uterus. Orgasm close to your delivery may start uterine contractions.

Many couples find that pregnancy poses new financial and emotional concerns that they hadn't anticipated. Those thoughts can come out in a number of ways, and may sometimes have unpleasant results. If you are physically abused while pregnant, your baby is also at risk of physical harm or death. The National Domestic Violence Hotline can link you to help in your area. A nationwide database includes detailed information on domestic violence shelters, legal advocacy, and assistance programs and social service programs. Call 1-800-799-SAFE. Remember, the greatest gift you can give your child is a happy, loving parent.

My last point is one you may need to keep in mind for a while. Your baby has gotten a lot from you. Her life, yes, and also maybe her eyes, her smile, maybe her nose and hair. You can also make sure she inherits your exercise habits.

From baby food, many children progress to sweetened breakfast cereals, and sweets are frequently used as a reward for good behavior. The baby everybody loves and thought so healthy and cute often grows up to be an adult who can't live without sugar and fat in his or her daily life. The result is a permanent weight problem that sets the stage for illness later in life.

Today, children's eating habits are shaped not only by their parents but also by advertising that makes junk food irresistibly appealing, and by society in general. Obesity is on the rise, and many children sooner consider having liposuction when they turn eighteen than exercising before that.

Tell your children that the reason you don't want them to eat sugars and junk food is because you love them and you want them to be strong and healthy. Invite them to work out with you, and instill good exercise beliefs in them early on. Remember, this is behavior, and behavior is reinforced by repetition until it becomes a habit.

That's all I have for you. Congratulations, again! I wish nothing but the best for you and your happy baby.